2005

Lives at Risk

Lives at Risk

Single-Payer National Health Insurance Around the World

John C. Goodman, Gerald L. Musgrave,
and Devon M. Herrick

Published in cooperation with the
National Center for Policy Analysis

ROWMAN & LITTLEFIELD PUBLISHERS, INC.
Lanham • Boulder • New York • Toronto • Oxford

ROWMAN & LITTLEFIELD PUBLISHERS, INC.

Published in the United States of America
by Rowman & Littlefield Publishers, Inc.
A wholly owned subsidary of The Rowman & Littlefield Publishing Group, Inc.
4501 Forbes Boulevard, Suite 200, Lanham, Maryland 20706
www.rowmanlittlefield.com

PO Box 317
Oxford
OX2 9RU, UK

British Library Cataloguing in Publication Information Available

Library of Congress Cataloging-in-Publication Data

Goodman, John C.
Lives at risk : single-payer national health insurance around the world / John C. Goodman, Gerald L.
Musgrave, and Devon M. Herrick.
    p. cm.
"Published in cooperation with the National Center for Policy Analysis."
Includes index.
ISBN 0-7425-4151-7 (cloth : alk. paper)— ISBN 0-7425-4152-5 (pbk. : alk. paper)
  1. National health insurance—Cross-cultural studies. 2. National health services—Cross-cultural
studies. 3. Medical policy—Cross-cultural studies. 4. Health care reform—United States.
5. Medical policy—United States.
  I. Single-Payer System. 2. Health Care Reform. 3. National Health Programs. 4. Program
Evaluation. I. Musgrave, Gerald L. II. Herrick, Devon M, 1963- III. National Center for Policy
Analysis (U.S.) IV. Title.

RA412.G66 2004
368.4'2—dc22   2004006468

Printed in the United States of America

Contents

Foreword

Bit by bit, we in the United States have been moving toward a system of health care in which the government assumes all responsibility for paying the bill—a single payer system. We took a major step in that direction with the enactment of Medicare and Medicaid in 1965 and narrowly avoided another major step with the rejection of the Clinton health plan in the early 1990s. At the end of World War II, government accounted for about 20 percent of all spending on health. This percentage has been rising ever since, slowly until 1965, then more rapidly after the advent of Medicare and Medicaid. Currently, government accounts for nearly half of all spending on health and almost surely for more than half if we include indirect spending through tax subsidies.

A single-payer system has great political appeal. It promises to provide quality health care to all, regardless of income, religion, race, or initial state of health. But does it live up to that promise? In this important book, John Goodman and his coauthors set out to find the answer. They examine health care in Canada, Britain, and New Zealand, three countries that have adopted national health insurance, and compare it with health care in the United States.

Their findings will surprise many and deserves wide attention.

Milton Friedman
Hoover Institution
April 3, 2004

Acknowledgments

The authors would like to thank the staff of the National Center for Policy Analysis who assisted in the preparation of this book. In particular, we thank Dorman Cordell, senior scholar, who edited the study that grew into this book; Donavan Wilson and Wess Mitchell, interns, who spent many hours checking references and verifying sources; Krishonne Johnson, publications manager, who created the graphics; Joe Barnett, director of publications, who helped edit the manuscript; Phyllis Guest, our copy editor; and Pam Dougherty, who proofed it.

We would also like to thank our reviewers: David Gratzer of the Manhattan Institute (New York City), John Graham of the Fraser Institute (Vancouver, Canada), Eamonn Butler of the Adam Smith Institute (London), and John Meadowcroft of the Institute of Economic Affairs (London). Their suggestions and critiques proved invaluable. Any errors of fact or omission are, of course, the responsibility of the authors.

Finally, we would also like to thank the staff of Rowman & Littlefield who have made this cooperative publishing venture possible.

Introduction: Thinking about Reform

As we move further into the twenty-first century, it is clear that we are living with a number of institutions that were not designed for the Information Age. One of those institutions is health care.

Virtually everyone agrees that our health care system needs reform. But what kind of reform? Some on the right would like to see us return to the type of system that prevailed in the 1950s. Some on the left would like to see us copy one of the government-run systems established in the mid-twentieth century and variously called socialized medicine, national health insurance and, more recently, single-payer health insurance. For example, Physicians for a National Health Program, claiming membership of 8,000 physicians and medical students, contends that "single-payer national health insurance would resolve virtually all of the major problems facing America's health care system today."[1]

We believe that neither of these two alternatives will work. But before we explain why, let us stop to consider some central problems that every reform faces. Most commentaries on health policy tend to ignore three very important facts about modern health systems:

1. We can potentially spend our entire gross domestic product (GDP) on health care in useful ways.
2. Whatever portion of our income we are spending on health care today, we are likely to want to spend more in the future.
3. We have suppressed normal market forces in dealing with characteristics one and two.

These facts are not in dispute. Rather, they are readily acknowledged by all health policy analysts. Also, the first two characteristics are not unique to health care. They are true of many other goods and services as well. But when combined with the third characteristic, they have devastating implications.

PROBLEM: OPPORTUNITIES TO SPEND MONEY ON HEALTH CARE ARE ALMOST UNLIMITED

Medical research has pushed the boundaries of what doctors can do for us in every direction. The Cooper Clinic in Dallas now offers an extensive checkup (with a full body scan) for about $1,500 or more.[2] Its clients include Ross Perot, Larry King, and other high-profile individuals. Yet, if everyone in America took advantage of this opportunity, we would increase our nation's annual health care bill by a third. More than 900 diagnostic tests can be done on blood alone,[3] and one doesn't need too much imagination to justify, say, $5,000 worth of tests each year. But if everyone did so, we would double the nation's health care bill. Americans purchase nonprescription drugs almost twelve billion times a year and almost all of these are acts of self-medication. Yet, if everyone sought a physician's advice before making such purchases, we would need twenty-five times the number of primary care physicians we currently have.[4] Some 1,100 tests can be done on our genes to determine if we have a predisposition toward one disease or another.[5] At, say, $1,000 a test, it would cost more than $1 million for a patient to run the full gamut. But if every American did so, the total cost would run to about thirty times the nation's total output of goods and services![6]

Notice that in hypothetically spending all of this money we have not yet cured a single disease or treated an actual illness. In these examples, we are simply collecting information. If in the process of the search we actually found something that warranted treatment, we could spend even more.

One of the cardinal beliefs of advocates of single-payer health insurance is that health care should be free at the point of consumption, regardless of willingness or ability to pay. But if health care really were free, people would have an incentive to obtain each and every service so long as it had any value to them. In other words, everybody would have at least an economic incentive to get the Cooper Clinic annual checkup, order dozens of blood tests, check out all their genes and consult physicians at the drop of a hat. In short order, unconstrained patients would attempt to spend the entire gross domestic product (GDP) on health care even though, as a practical matter, that would be impossible.

"Free" health care is of course not really free. It is care paid directly by employers, government or some other entity, and indirectly by workers and taxpayers. The more employers pay for health care the less employees receive in wages. The more the government pays, the less after-tax income taxpayers have. Therefore, allowing patients to go on an unconstrained shopping spree in the medical marketplace would ultimately impoverish all of us.

No serious person wants this result. Not even the advocates of single-payer health insurance want it. Instead, they envision placing many obstacles in the path of patients and doctors in order to constrain spending. These obstacles may not be prices, but they most certainly involve costs, such as the cost of waiting for care. Although its advocates call national health insurance "single-payer insurance" these days, its distinguishing characteristic is not control of demand. It is control of supply.

Like the systems of Canada and Britain, American health maintenance organizations (HMOs) also make health care free to their enrollees at the point of delivery. They then control access to care, especially expensive care, on a case-by-case basis. Whether or not an HMO patient gets an MRI brain scan, for example, depends upon the symptoms and the probable outcome of the scan, as well as its cost. HMOs, therefore, control costs by curtailing demand.

Nothing like that happens in countries with national health insurance, however. For one thing, doctors in Canada would have no idea how much a scan actually costs and therefore would have no basis for comparing costs with probable medical benefits. The number of brain scans is controlled in Canada, not on the basis of a case-by-case review of patient conditions, but because of spending constraints to limit the number of MRI scanners.

Many American doctors have endorsed the single-payer idea, in part because they envy the ability of Canadian doctors to practice medicine without managed-care-type, third-party interference. What they overlook is that, at least from a budget perspective, Canadian officials have no reason to care what decisions doctors make. They limit the number of scanners, and therefore the expense of scanning, before doctors see even a single patient. American physicians who support single-payer insurance also tend to discount lack of access to expensive diagnostic equipment in Canada, believing that the problem could be ameliorated by just spending more. They do not realize that the only reason the Canadian system works at all is because the government controls supply. If Canadian doctors (who, again, have no idea what anything costs) had access to an unlimited supply of MRI units, they might spend Canada's entire GDP on brain scans!

In general, countries with national health insurance control costs by imposing arbitrary limits. They strictly control the number of doctors who can be specialists. They limit access to modern medical technology. The more expensive the service, the more difficult they make access. As a result, in countries with national health insurance, people wait. They wait in the offices of general practitioners. They wait to see specialists. They wait for surgeries. And waiting is a rationing device comparable to money prices in a market system.

In this book we will stress many differences between the U.S. health care system and government-run health care systems. But on the demand side, the differences are not as great as one might suppose. Although health care is not free at the point of consumption for the average American, it is almost free. On the average, every time a patient spends a dollar on hospital care in our country, only two cents comes out of the patient's own pocket. The other ninety-eight cents is paid by a third party (an employer, insurer or government.). On the average, for every dollar patients spend on physician care, only twelve cents comes out of their own pockets. And for the health care system as a whole, patients pay directly only eighteen cents of every dollar they spend. The rest is spent by some other entity.[7]

On the demand side, the problem with a system with no money prices is that people view each good or service as though its price were zero. As a result, they tend to try to consume the item so long as it has any value at all. The problem this creates is enormous waste. People seek services until the value to them is almost zero, even though the cost of these services may be quite high. The upshot is that people consume services for which the social benefit is well below the social cost. In Britain, for example, people have to pay out of pocket to see a movie, go to the theater or witness a sporting event. But the only costs to see a physician are the costs of travel and waiting time. So although the government makes an enormous investment in their training, British physicians spend an inordinate amount of time on trivial complaints.

In the United States, things are not that much better. Although no one wants to enter a hospital, once there, the typical patient in this country has an incentive to use hospital services until they are worth only two cents at the margin (or about 1/50th of the actual cost). Aside from the costs of time and travel and the risk of being around other sick people, patients have an incentive to utilize physicians' services until they are worth only twelve cents on the dollar. And for the health care system as a whole, our incentive is to spend until the services we receive are worth only eighteen cents on the dollar. No wonder there is so much waste!

In principle, there are not many solutions to this problem. Someone must choose between health care and other uses of money. The question is, who will that someone be? The answer of single-payer advocates is medical bureaucracies answerable to politicians. And much of this book will be spent looking in some detail at how rationing decisions are made in these systems.

A second method for choosing between health care and other uses of money is the method of managed care. The paradigm is the HMO. As noted above, HMOs have far less rationing by waiting than do national health insurance schemes. One reason for the difference is that HMOs tend to make rationing decisions based on medical and economic rather than political considerations. Because some policy analysts believe that a system of competing managed care organizations can solve the problems of single-payer health insurance, we devote a chapter to that idea.

The third method of choosing between health care and other uses of money is to allow patients themselves to choose. A vehicle that facilitates such choices is a health savings account (HSA), from which patients pay medical expenses directly. Funds not spent on health care grow in the account and may be used for other purposes. Singapore has had a compulsory system of "medisave" accounts since 1984.[8] Medical savings accounts (MSAs) were introduced in South Africa in the early 1990s and today represent 65 percent of the market for private health insurance in that country.[9] The United States experimented with a pilot program for several years and as of January 1, 2004, HSAs are available to all nonelderly Americans.[10]

So far, these accounts have mainly been used to pay relatively small medical bills, less than a few thousand dollars. These are the expenses that fall under a health insurance deductible. But as the accounts grow and if health insurance evolves toward the casualty model, the accounts could play a role in almost every aspect of health care. Consider homeowner's casualty insurance, for example. If hail damages a roof, an insurance adjuster surveys the damage and agrees to a sum sufficient to cover the cost of repair—usually by a repair service the insurer knows. But the homeowner is not restricted to this option. He or she can choose other, more expensive repair services or even choose to replace the damaged roof with a nicer roof.

In principle, health insurance could work the same way. In the case of expensive heart surgery or cancer care, the insurer could direct the patient to a hospital or clinic and agree to pay the full cost. But the patient would be free to take the same reimbursement amount and apply it to another hospital or clinic, paying any extra charges from an HSA account.

In the world of casualty insurance, auto repair shops act as agents of automobile owners. Roofing repair services act as agents of homeowners. Suppliers of these services do not see themselves as agents of third-party insurers. In a similar way, HSAs could free patients to become the real decision makers, choosing between health care and other uses of money in virtually every part of the health care system. In such a world, doctors, nurses and other providers would see themselves as agents of their patients rather than agents of impersonal bureaucracies.

PROBLEM: THE DESIRE TO
SPEND WILL GROW IN THE FUTURE

Let's now turn to a second well-documented, but rarely discussed, fact about modern health care systems. Whatever we are spending on health care today, we are probably going to want to spend more tomorrow. This is true for two reasons: first, the average age in all developed countries is rising and health needs increase with age, and second, health care is a "superior good," which means as income grows people choose to spend more of it on health care.

At 15.2 percent of the GDP, the United States spends more of its income on health care than any other nation, a sum that equals $1.6 trillion.[11] This fact is a usual source of criticism both at home and abroad. But if you think 15 percent is high, you haven't seen anything yet. Currently, senior citizens (over sixty-five years of age) spend about 45 percent of all their consumption (regardless of who pays for it) on medical care. By 2020, it is estimated that three-fourths of all consumption by seniors will be on health care.

Is such spending good or bad? That depends on whether people are getting their money's worth for the dollars they spend. If people are getting value for money, nothing is wrong with devoting more resources to health care. If they are not getting value for money, something *is* wrong with it.

This way of looking at the issue is very different from what one hears in most public policy discussions. The standard complaint is that health care "costs" are rising. And innumerable conferences, briefings, books, articles, essays and so forth have sought to "solve the problem" of rising health care costs.

Note that in a general sense "spending" and "costs" are the same thing. If people are aging and their incomes are rising, one can predict with great confidence that they will want to devote more of their income to medical care. Not only is this not a "problem," it is a natural and inevitable part of life. Indeed, to the degree that this phenomenon is viewed as a problem, it is not a problem that is going to be solved. It will only get worse through time.

We noted above that in a system with no prices, decision makers cannot determine what value people place on different services. Thus, they cannot know what's being oversupplied or undersupplied. A similar problem arises with respect to total spending on health care. Given that it should rise over time, by how much should it rise? How would one know? Without markets through which people can reveal their preferences for health care versus other goods and services, it's anybody's guess.

American employers who complain about the "problem" of rising health care costs are in a similar situation. Because decisions about health care typically are made collectively at the workplace and because the premiums employees pay rarely reflect real costs, employers have no way of discerning their employees' willingness to trade off higher wages for more health care, except through union negotiations and other imperfect devices. Fortunately, when American employers make a mistake, its consequences are confined to their companies and their workforces. But when the managers of national health insurance make mistakes, the whole nation suffers.

PROBLEM: WE HAVE SUPPRESSED
NORMAL MARKET RESPONSES

Some of the things we have been saying about health care are also true of other goods and services. For example, we could probably spend our entire gross domestic product on automobiles, with each of us owning several to use over different terrains and in different seasons. But no one ever asserts that this is a problem. To the contrary, most people regard it as an opportunity. The fact that automobile manufacturers have discovered so many different ways to satisfy our needs makes us better off, not worse off (pollution problems aside).

Similarly, fine wine is probably a superior good. As people's income rises, they tend to buy more of it. And in recent years, supply has increased to meet demand, as vineyards have expanded all over the world. Again, no one regards this as a problem.

So what makes automobiles and fine wine different from health care? Why are problems that cause so much hand-wringing in health care not seen as problems in the other two markets? The answer is that in this country and in all developed countries we have suppressed the ability of the market to allocate health care resources.

The suppression of the market in health care began more than 100 years ago. It started with controls on who could be a physician and how those licensed to practice should behave. By the mid-twentieth century, controls were extended to the hospital sector and then to health insurance. By the 1970s, with government paying more and more medical bills, policy makers realized that prices and markets were not able to do their job. Similar trends occurred in other developed countries.[12]

What does it mean to suppress normal market forces in health care? Not long ago, if a doctor competed aggressively against other doctors, say, the way auto companies compete against each other, he or she could be in real trouble. For example, if the doctor posted his normal fees and compared them to other doctors' fees, if he compared the quality of his practice to that of another physician or if he advertised at all he could be expelled from the county medical society. That, in turn, would lead to a loss of privileges at all the hospitals in his area. If the offense were bad enough (irritating enough to his fellow physicians), he could lose his license to practice medicine.

Until very recently, the hospital sector was dominated by nonprofit institutions whose sole task was to facilitate the doctors' goal of treating patients. Not only were hospitals not supposed to function like businesses, they went out of their way to avoid certain common business practices. For example, for a hospital to compare the quality of its care to the quality offered by a competitor would have been unthinkable. Advertising itself was unthinkable. Not only did hospitals not post their prices, no one paid them other than the occasional uninsured patient. At the time Medicare (for seniors) and Medicaid (for the poor) were adopted in the 1960s, virtually every hospital in the United States was paid by insurers based on cost-plus reimbursement. And when the federal government set up Medicare, it joined the cost-plus system, paying for health care the way it paid for weapons systems. All in all, the health care system in this country and throughout the developed world functioned according to rules that resembled a medieval guild more than a complex modern market.[13]

Times have changed. And they have changed more in the United States than anywhere else. Other countries have left in place the medieval guild approach to medicine and tried to control costs in crude ways that we will examine. In this country, however, we have made dismantling the guild and promoting competition a public policy goal.

Doctors today can compete in almost any way they like. They can post prices; they can advertise; they can boast about the quality of care they deliver. Hospitals can do the same. And insurers can pay hospitals based on any arrangement that can be reached through a no-holds-barred voluntary exchange in the marketplace. But although the shackles have been removed and the law no longer protects it, the 100-year-old culture that has dominated medical practice has not disappeared.

Pick up almost any daily newspaper and you will find evidence that the medical marketplace is still not functioning like other markets. "Hospitals Say They are Penalized by Medicare for Improving Care," blares a front page headline in the *New York Times*.[14] "More Medicine Is Not Better Medicine," leads a *Times* guest editorial, citing evidence that Medicare spends twice as much on seniors in Manhattan as it does in Portland, Oregon, without getting any improvement in quality or patient satisfaction.[15]

But there are two consoling observations: first, the medical marketplace is becoming more competitive, and second, things are much worse in every other country.

HAVE OTHER COUNTRIES FOUND THE ANSWER?

American advocates of single-payer national health insurance propose to[16]

- Eliminate HMOs and most other forms of managed care
- Have all health care financed by the government, with no premiums or co-payments from those covered
- Control costs by assigning global budgets to hospitals and setting fees and salaries for physicians
- Prohibit private insurance or personal payment for any service covered by the single-payer system

In advancing this idea, they point to other countries as examples of health care systems that are superior to our own. Are they right?

The promise of national health insurance is that government will make health care available on the basis of need rather than ability to pay. That implies a government commitment to meet health care needs. It implies that rich and poor will have equal access to care. And it implies that more serious needs will be given priority over the less serious. Unfortunately, these promises have not been kept.

- Wherever national health insurance has been tried, rationing by waiting is pervasive—with waits that force patients to endure pain and sometimes put their lives at risk.
- Not only is access to health care not equal, if anything it tends to correlate with income—with the middle class getting more access than the poor and the rich getting more access than the middle class, especially when income classes are weighted by incidence of illness.
- Not only are health care resources not allocated on the basis of need, these systems tend to overspend on the relatively healthy while denying the truly sick access to specialist care and lifesaving medical technology.
- And far from establishing national priorities that get care first to those who need it most, these systems leave rationing choices up to local bureaucracies that, for example, fill hospital beds with chronic patients while acute patients wait for care.

It might seem that some of these problems could be easily remedied. Yet, as the years of failed reform efforts in Britain and Canada have shown, the defects of single-payer systems of national health insurance are not easily remedied. The reason: the characteristics described above are not accidental byproducts of government-run health care systems. They are the natural and inevitable consequences of placing the health care market under the control of politicians.[17] It is not true that health care policies in countries with single-payer health insurance just happen to be what they are. In most cases, they could not be otherwise.

Why do single-payer health insurance schemes skimp on expensive services to the seriously ill while providing so many inexpensive services to the marginally ill? Because the latter services benefit millions of people (read: millions of voters), while acute and intensive care services concentrate large amounts of money on a handful of patients (read: small numbers of voters). Democratic political pressures dictate the redistribution of resources from the few to the many.

Why are sensitive rationing decisions and other issues of hospital management left to hospital bureaucracies? As a practical matter, no government can make it a national policy to let 25,000 of its citizens die from lack of the best cancer treatment every year, as apparently happens in Britain.[18] Nor can any government announce that some people must wait for surgery so that the elderly can use hospitals as nursing homes or that elderly patients must be moved so that surgery can proceed. These decisions are so emotionally loaded that no elected official could afford to claim responsibility for them. Important decisions on who will receive care and how that care will be delivered are left to the hospital bureaucracy because no other course is politically possible.

Why do low-income patients fare so poorly under national health insurance? Because such insurance is almost always a middle-class phenomenon. Prior to its introduction, every country had some government-funded program to meet the health care needs of the poor. The middle-class working population not only paid for its own health care, but also paid taxes to fund health care for the poor. Single-payer health insurance extends the "free ride" to those who pay taxes to support it. Such systems respond to the political demands of the middle-class population and serve the interests of this population.

Why do the rich and the powerful manage to jump the queues and obtain care that is denied to others? Because it could not be otherwise. These are the people with the power to change the system. If members of Parliament had to wait in line for their care like ordinary people, the system would not last for a minute.

DO OTHER COUNTRIES THINK THEY HAVE FOUND THE ANSWER?

Despite the official rhetoric, over the course of the past decade almost every European country with a national health care system has introduced market-oriented reforms and turned to the private sector to reduce the costs of care and increase the value, availability and effectiveness of treatments.[19] In making these changes, more often than not these countries looked to the United States for guidance.

- About seven million people in Britain now have private health insurance; and since the Labor government assumed power, the number of patients paying out of pocket for medical treatment has increased by 40 percent.[20]
- To reduce its waiting lists, the British National Health Service (NHS) recently announced that it will treat some patients in private hospitals, reversing a long-standing policy of using only public hospitals;[21] and, the NHS has even contracted with HCA International, America's largest health care provider, to treat 10,000 NHS cancer patients at its facilities in Britain.
- Australia has turned to the private sector to reform its public health care system to such an extent that it is now second only to the United States among industrialized nations in the share of health care spending that is private.[22]
- Since 1993, the German government has experimented with American-style managed competition by giving Germans the right to choose among the country's competing sickness funds (insurers).[23]
- The Netherlands also has American-style managed competition, with an extensive network of private health care providers and slightly more than one-third of the population insured privately.[24]
- Sweden is introducing reforms that will allow private providers to deliver more than 40 percent of all health care services and about 80 percent of primary care in Stockholm.[25]
- Even Canada has changed, using the United States as a partial safety valve for its overtaxed health care system; provincial governments and patients spend more than $1 billion a year on U.S. medical care.[26]

In each of these countries, growing frustration with government health programs has led to a reexamination of the fundamental principles of health care delivery. Through bitter experience, many of the countries that once touted the benefits of government control have learned that the surest remedy for their countries' health care crises is not increasing government power, but increasing patient power instead.[27]

GOAL OF THIS BOOK

This book is not intended as a defense of the existing health care system in the United States. To the contrary, we count ourselves among its harshest critics.

Our goal here is to dispel certain myths about health care as delivered in countries that have national health insurance. These myths have gained the status of fact in both the United States and abroad, even though the evidence shows a far different reality.

In this book we will examine the critical failures of national health insurance systems without focusing on minor blemishes or easily correctable problems. In doing so, our goal is to identify the problems common to all countries with national health insurance and to explain why these problems emerge. Most national health care systems are in a state of sustained internal crisis as costs rise and the stated goals of universal access and quality care are not met. In almost all cases, the reason is the same: the politics of medicine. The problems of government-run health care systems flow inexorably from the fact that they are government-run rather than market driven.

We have chosen to focus primarily, though not exclusively, on the health care systems of English-speaking countries whose cultures are similar to our own. Britain, Canada and New Zealand in particular are often pointed to by advocates of national health insurance as models for U.S. health care system reform. In amassing evidence of how these systems actually work, many of our sources are government publications or commentary and analysis by reporters and scholars who fully support the concept of socialized medicine.

The failure of national health insurance is a secret of modern social science. Not only have scholars failed to understand the defects of national health insurance, too often advocates and ordinary citizens hold an idealized view of it. For that reason, we present much of the information in the form of rebuttals to commonly held myths.[28]

NOTES

1. Don R. McCanne, "Would Single-Payer Health Insurance Be Good for America?" *Physicians for a National Health Program* (March 27, 2000).

2. Information available at www.cooperaerobics.com/clinic.

3. John C. Goodman and Gerald L. Musgrave, *Patient Power: Solving America's Health Care Crisis* (Washington, D.C.: Cato Institute, 1992), 79.

4. Simon Rottenberg, "Unintended Consequences: The Probable Effects of Mandated Medical Insurance," *Regulation* 13, no. 2 (Summer 1990): 27–28.

5. Michael Walholz, "Genetic Testing Hits the Doctor's Office" *Wall Street Journal*, December 3, 2003.

6. The calculations are thus: the U.S. population of 288.4 million people multiplied by $1.1 million per capita for the battery of tests. The resulting figure of $317.2 trillion dollars is approximately 28.67 times the fourth quarter 2003 (annualized) gross domestic product of $11 trillion.

7. U.S. Department of Health and Human Services, "Distribution of Health Care Expenses, 1996," Medical Expenditure Panel Survey, Highlights, no. 11, AHRQ Pub. No. 00-0024, U.S. Department of Health and Human Services, May 2000.

8. Thomas A. Massaro and Yu-Ning Wong, "Medical Savings Accounts: The Singapore Experience," National Center for Policy Analysis, NCPA Policy Report No. 203, April 1996.

9. Shaun Matisonn, "Medical Savings Accounts in South Africa," National Center for Policy Analysis, Policy Report No. 234, June 2000.

10. Greg Scandlen, "MSAs Can Be a Windfall for All," National Center for Policy Analysis, NCPA Policy Backgrounder, No. 157, November 2, 2001. The Prescription Drug and Medicare Modernization Act of 2003 created a new type of personal health account that is available to 250 million (nonelderly) Americans and is called a health savings account (HSA). See Greg Scandlen, "Health Savings Accounts Will Empower All Americans," Galen Institute, December 3, 2003.

11. Stephen Heffler et al., "Health Spending Projections for 2002–2012," *Health Affairs* (February 7, 2003) (Web exclusive).

12. John C. Goodman, *The Regulation of Medical Care: Is the Price Too High?* (San Francisco, Calif.: Cato Institute, 1980).

13. See Goodman and Musgrave, *Patient Power*, ch. 5.

14. Reed Abelson, "Hospitals Say They Are Penalized by Medicare for Improving Care," *New York Times*, December 5, 2003.

15. Elliott S. Fisher, "More Medicine Is Not Better Medicine," *New York Times*, December 1, 2003.

16. See Physicians' Working Group on Single-Payer National Health Insurance, "Proposal for Health Care Reform," May 1, 2001.

17. John C. Goodman and Philip K. Porter, "Political Equilibrium and the Provision of Public Goods," *Public Choice*, forthcoming.

18. Karol Sikora, "Cancer Survival in Britain," *British Medical Journal* (August 21, 1999): 461–62.

19. Marshall W. Raffel, *Health Care and Reform in Industrialized Countries* (University Park, Pa.: The University of Pennsylvania Press, 1997). Also see Monique Jérôme-Forget, Joseph White and Joshua M. Wiener, *Health Care Reform through Internal Markets: Experience and Proposal* (Washington, D.C.: Brookings Institution Press, 1995); and Wendy Ranade, ed., *Markets and Health Care: A Comparative Analysis* (New York: Longman, 1998).

20. "Thousands Shun the NHS," *BBC Health,* March 2000. Another one million people have taken out cash-benefit critical illness insurance. See Oliver Wright, "Private Health Cover Slumps as Cost Spirals," *The Times*, September 17, 2003.

21. "UK to Strike New Deal with Private Health Sector," *Reuters Health,* December 4, 2001.

22. Organization for Economic Cooperation and Development, *OECD Health Data 2000* (Paris: OECD, 2000).

23. For a discussion of managed competition in Germany, see Stefan Greg, Kieke Okma and Franz Hessel, "Managed Competition in Health Care in the Netherlands and Germany—Theoretical Foundation, Empirical Findings and Policy Conclusion,"

Lehrstuhl für Allgemeine Betriebswirtschaftslehre und Gesundheitsmanagement der Ernst-Moritz-Arndt-Universität Greifswald, Diskussionspapier, April/May 2001.

24. Kieke Okma, "Health Care, Health Policies and Health Care Reforms in the Netherlands," School of Public Policy Studies, Queen's University, Kingston, Ontario, March 2000.

25. Johan Hjertqvist, "Swedish Health-Care Reform: From Public Monopolies to Market Services," Montreal Economic Institute, 2001, available at www.iedm.org/library/Hjertqvist_en.html.

26. Victor Dirnfeld, "The Benefits of Privatization," *Canadian Medical Association Journal* 155, no. 4 (August 15, 1996): 407–10. For instance, many Canadian provinces now send breast cancer and prostate cancer patients to the United States for radiation therapy. For a discussion of Canadian cancer patients' being sent to the U.S. for radiation treatment, see Mark Cardwell, "Quebec Cancer Patients to Head South," *Medical Post* 35, no. 22 (June 8, 1999); Robert Walker, "Alberta Centre May Soon Fly Its CA Patients South," *Medical Post* 35, no. 34 (October 12, 1999); Lynn Haley et al., "Guarding the Border," *Medical Post* 36, no. 01 (January 4, 2000); and Doug Brunk, "Canada Sends Overflow of CA Patients Down South," *Family Practice News* (May 1, 2000).

27. Task Force Report, *An Agenda for Solving America's Health Care Crisis*, National Center for Policy Analysis, Policy Report No. 151, May 1990; and Goodman and Musgrave, *Patient Power.*

28. The "Myths" section is an expanded and completely updated version of a study published by the National Center for Policy Analysis in 1991: John C. Goodman and Gerald L. Musgrave, "Twenty Myths about National Health Insurance," National Center for Policy Analysis, Policy Report No. 128, December 1991.

Part One

TWENTY MYTHS

Chapter One

Rights

MYTH NO. 1: IN COUNTRIES WITH SINGLE-PAYER NATIONAL HEALTH CARE SYSTEMS, PEOPLE HAVE A RIGHT TO HEALTH CARE

"Access to comprehensive health care is a human right," according to the U.S. Physicians' Working Group for Single-Payer National Health Insurance. "It is the responsibility of society, through its government, to ensure this right."[1] Virtually every government that has established a system of national health insurance has proclaimed health care to be a basic human right.

In fact, there is no such right in any sense that people ordinarily understand the meaning of the term. What the right to care means almost everywhere is nothing more than the opportunity to get services for free (or at very little cost) as the government decides to make those services available. But government is under no obligation to provide any particular service. And if it fails to provide a service, people are not entitled to go to court and sue the way that Americans, for example, can sue an employer, a health maintenance organization (HMO) or even Medicaid.

Citizens of Canada, for example, have no right to any particular health care service. They have no right to an MRI scan. They have no right to heart surgery. They do not even have the right to a place in line. The 100th person waiting for heart surgery is not entitled to the 100th surgery. Other people can and do jump the queue. In fact, in the 1980s some Canadian hospitals advertised in America in search of paying customers to help out with their cash-strapped budgets. Yet, it was illegal for Canadian citizens to pay for the same services. Canadian hospitals and doctors are not allowed to accept money from Canadian patients for any medical services covered by their single-payer system, nor are private insurers allowed to cover such services.[2]

Although the practice has since been discontinued, in part because of public embarrassment, for awhile one could maintain that Americans had more rights in the Canadian health care system than Canadians did. More recently, American members of Toronto professional sports teams were jumping the queue by paying for care at Ontario hospitals. A new law outlaws this practice as well.[3] One could even argue that Canadians have fewer rights than their pets. While Canadian pet owners can purchase an MRI scan for their cat or dog, purchasing a scan for themselves is illegal (although more and more human patients are finding legal loopholes, as we shall see below).[4]

Canada is not alone. We know of no country in the world that has established a universal right to any particular health care service. The one exception is the United States. Unlike countries with national health insurance, the United States grants every citizen a legally enforceable right (entitlement) to kidney dialysis treatment at government expense.

As noted in the introduction, countries with single-payer health insurance limit health care spending by limiting supply. They do so primarily by imposing global budgets on hospitals and area health authorities. Often there is a separate budget for high-tech equipment, to make doubly sure that high-cost procedures are curtailed.[5] The consequence of making health care free, thus creating unconstrained demand, while limiting supply is that demand exceeds supply for virtually every service. That, in turn, leads to rationing, usually by forcing patients to wait for treatment.

By U.S. standards, rationing by waiting is one of the cruelest aspects of government-run health care systems.[6] How much waiting is there? That is not an easy question to answer. Since waiting is viewed by most governments as an embarrassment, public officials are reluctant to collect and publish information about it. However, some facts are available:

- In England, with a population of almost sixty million, government statistics show more than one million are waiting to be admitted to hospitals at any one time.[7]
- In Canada, with a population of more than thirty-one million, the independent Fraser Institute found that more than 876,584 are waiting for treatment of all types.[8]
- In Norway, with a population of almost 4.5 million, 270,000 are waiting in queues on any given day for various types of medical treatments, including hospital admission.[9]
- In New Zealand, with a population of about 3.6 million, the government reports the number of people on waiting lists for surgery and other treatments is more than 90,000.[10]

On the surface, the number of people waiting may seem small relative to the total population, ranging from 0.5 percent in Canada to around 2.5 percent in New Zealand. However, considering that only 16 percent of the population enters a hospital each year in developed countries and that only a small percent requires serious (and expensive) procedures, these numbers are quite high.[11] In New Zealand, if 11 percent (496,000) are admitted to a hospital each year, a waiting list of 90,000 would represent a ratio of almost one person waiting for every five who receive treatment.

Patients may wait for months or even years for treatment.[12] For example:

- Canadian patients waited an average of 8.3 weeks in 2003 from the time they were referred to a specialist until the actual consultation, and another 9.5 weeks before treatment, including surgery.[13]
- In New Zealand, the average waiting time for elderly patients in need of hip or knee replacement is 300 and 400 days, respectively, and many wait much longer.[14]
- Of the 90,000 people waiting for surgery or treatment in New Zealand in 1997, more than 20,000 waited for a period of more than two years.[15]
- In Britain, 43,900 patients, many of them needing hip or knee replacements, had been waiting for more than a year at the end of 2001.[16]
- The London-based Adam Smith Institute estimates the people currently on the NHS waiting lists will collectively wait about one million years longer to receive treatment than doctors deem acceptable.[17]

Official lists often understate the length of the wait because a given treatment might require waiting in more than one queue. For instance, a Canadian patient must initially see a general practitioner (GP) for a referral to a specialist. The patient may then wait weeks or months to see that specialist. After the specialist's examination, a patient usually faces another wait for treatment. In many cases, a given treatment involves several waits—a wait for a diagnostic test and another for surgery, for example.[18]

Figure 1.1 shows the average length of time Canadian patients wait from the time they are referred by a GP to the time of actual treatment. As the figure shows, waiting times are long all across Canada and they vary considerably from province to province. They range, for example, from a low of 14.3 weeks in Ontario, on the average, to almost seven months in Saskatchewan. Figure 1.2 shows waiting times by specialty. Again, the waits are long for all treatments, and they range from 6.1 weeks, on the average, for cancer (medical oncology) treatment to more than seven months for orthopedic surgery.

Note also that waiting times increased during the 1990s in every province and for every type of procedure. As we shall see below, advocates of single-payer health insurance claim that Canada has been more successful than the

FIGURE 1-1

Numbers of Weeks Patients Wait between Referral by GP and Treatment, by Province, in Canada

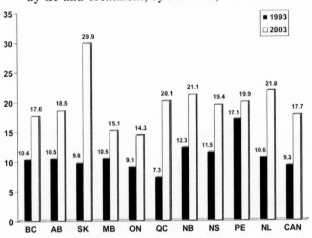

Note: Median waiting times. The Canadian provinces are: British Columbia, Alberta, Saskatchewan, Manitoba, Ontario, Quebec, New Brunswick, Nova Scotia, Prince Edward Island, and Newfoundland.

Source: Nadeem Esmail and Michael Walker. "Waiting Your Turn: Hospital Waiting Lists in Canada, 13th Edition," Fraser Institute, Critical Issues Bulletin, October 2003; Cynthia Ramsay and Michael Walker, "Waiting Your Turn: Hospital Waiting Lists in Canada, 7th Edition," Fraser Institute, Critical Issues Bulletin, 1997.

FIGURE 1-2

Numbers of Weeks Patients Wait between Referral by GP and Treatment, by Specialty, in Canada

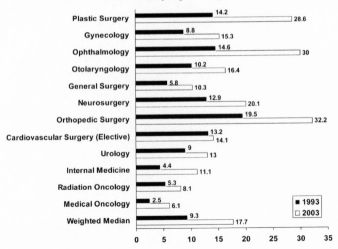

Note: Median waiting times.

Source: Nadeem Esmail and Michael Walker, "Waiting Your Turn: Hospital Waiting Lists in Canada, 13th Edition," Fraser Institute, Critical Issues Bulletin, October 2003; Cynthia Ramsay and Michael Walker, "Waiting Your Turn: Hospital Waiting Lists in Canada, 7th Edition," Fraser Institute, Critical Issues Bulletin, 1997.

United States at holding down health care costs. This success, however, has come at a very heavy price for patients.

In Britain, although the National Health Service (NHS) claims that more than 95 percent of patients are treated within twelve months, many are not.[19] The most recent NHS records show that 22,182 patients had been waiting for treatment between twelve and seventeen months—less than half the 46,333 on waiting lists a mere nine months earlier.[20] However, the NHS is now manipulating the system by identifying and treating patients up against the twelve-month limit to make its statistics look better, even though average waiting times for patients with serious conditions have not necessarily been reduced.[21] Also, Britain's National Audit Office, which scrutinizes public spending on behalf of Parliament, reports that many health authorities have made "inappropriate adjustments" to make their waiting lists appear smaller.[22] As one critic observed, "If a number becomes politically important, it becomes unreliable. The easier it is to manipulate the figures, the quicker this will be done. This is as true of the budget as of NHS waiting lists."[23]

Patients queuing for treatment in single-payer countries are often waiting in pain. Many are risking their lives. An investigation by a British newspaper, *The Observer*, finds that delays in Britain for colon cancer treatment are so long that 20 percent of the cases considered curable at time of diagnosis are incurable by the time of treatment.[24] A study of cancer patients in Glasgow, Scotland, finds the same is true of lung cancer patients.[25] Twenty-five percent of British cardiac patients die while waiting their turn to receive treatment.[26] According to government reports, one in six people on NHS waiting lists for elective surgery are removed without ever being treated.[27]

During one twelve-month period, 121 patients in Ontario, Canada, were removed from a waiting list for coronary bypass surgery because they had become too sick to undergo surgery with a reasonable risk of survival.[28] A study for Health Canada, the federal health agency that oversees the Health Canada Act, says government waiting lists may be inflated "20 percent to 30 percent" by the presence of patients "who have already received the procedure, have died, never knew they were on a list," and so on. The government defends these practices as evidence of efficiency, saying, "Waiting is widely associated with publicly funded health care systems; it indicates the absence of costly excess capacity."[29] That is an understatement.

Sometimes patients on waiting lists seek treatment in other countries. As we shall see below, Canadians occasionally cross the border into the United States to obtain care they cannot get in Canada. Sometimes Canadian provinces even pay for the treatment. Until recently, British patients were allowed to seek reimbursed treatment abroad under special circumstances. For example, in 2000, the NHS sent 1,100 Britons to continental European hospitals for treatment.

Many of the procedures were hip replacements and cataract surgeries for people who had waited for long periods.[30] An additional 200 Britons sought permission for treatment on the continent, but were turned down by their local health authorities.[31]

In a British Consumers' Association survey, more than half of those polled thought the NHS should pay for treatment abroad if it could be provided more quickly and more cheaply than in Britain.[32] The British government has resisted that option.[33] Today, the Norwegian government sends patients who have been waiting for extended periods to other countries for treatment by doctors with private practices, in private hospitals.[34] European courts have twice ruled that refusing reimbursement for cross-border medical treatment violates the free movement of goods guaranteed by the Treaty of Rome, which governs the European Union. Due to these decisions, Britons, like other Europeans, will be more likely in the future to shop for health care in other EU countries to avoid long waiting lines at home.[35]

Although crossing a border to obtain health care is not yet common in Europe,[36] many governments are justifiably worried that patients will seek care elsewhere due to perceived or real differences in quality. Also, spending on health care is limited in all European countries, but there are different degrees of rationing for different services in different countries. If patients were able to cross borders at will for treatment, they could potentially circumvent any waiting list. Mobility could create an artificial market for health care, one in which waiting times tend to equalize across countries—much as prices tend to equalize in competitive markets. Also, this type of patient migration would defeat many of the attempts by single-payer countries to control health spending.

RATIONING IN THE UNITED STATES

There is also rationing of care in the United States, more than many people may realize. This is especially true in public hospitals that provide care to the uninsured and in Medicare (for the elderly) and Medicaid (for the poor). These government programs face many of the same political pressures as national health insurance systems. For example:

- Doctors estimate that as many as half of the 300,000 people on dialysis in the United States might benefit from six-day-a-week treatment; but because Medicare covers a maximum of three days a week, only a few hundred patients receive the more extensive treatment.[37]
- Only about one in fifteen patients who could benefit from it gets a new device called HeartMate because Medicare will not pay the full cost; by one

estimate, Medicare would have to pay $15 to $20 billion a year to furnish one to every patient who needs it.[38]

- Eli Lilly and Company makes the drug Xigris to treat severe sepsis, a disease that kills 250,000 people a year; but because Medicare balks at paying its steep cost—$6,800 a treatment—doctors wrote fewer than 15,000 prescriptions for the drug in 2002, although 750,000 people suffer from sepsis each year.[39]
- On the other hand, Medicare does pay for colonoscopies and because the procedure has enjoyed a surge in popularity, demand has far outstripped supply, causing patients in some parts of the country to wait for months.[40]

In defense of its practices, Medicare claims that some of these expensive therapies are of unproven value. But the same claim is often made in defense of rationing by the governments of other countries.

In a recent survey of U.S. hospitals, 98 percent admitted to some rationing of MRI scans, 8 percent rationed PET imaging scans,[41] 27 percent rationed the drug Xigris, and 35 percent admitted to some rationing of access to intensive care units.[42] How does the U.S. experience compare to that of other countries? A study by the Commonwealth Fund and Harvard School of Public Health found that only about 5 percent of Americans undergoing surgery have to wait more than four months. As figure 1.3 shows, the comparable figure is

FIGURE 1-3

Patients Having to Wait More Than Four Months for Surgery[1]

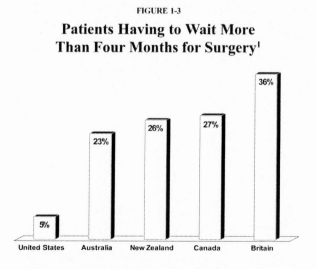

[1] Percent of all adult surgery patients receiving elective (nonemergency) surgery in last two years.

Source: Cathy Schoen, Robert J. Blendon, Catherine M. DesRoches, and Robin Osborn, "Comparison of Health Care System Views and Experiences in Five Nations, 2001," Commonwealth Fund, Issue Brief, May 2002.

26 percent or more in New Zealand and Canada and more than 36 percent in Britain.

Granted that rationing in the United States is not as bad as rationing in other countries, are the differences mere differences of degree, or are they also differences of kind? Our evidence will show that there are differences of kind.

NOTES

1. Steffie Woolhandler et al., "Proposal of the Physicians' Working Group for Single-Payer National Health Insurance," *Journal of the American Medical Association* vol. 290, no. 6 (August 13, 2003), 798–805.

2. Canadian provinces and territories set up their own health programs in the years following World War II. Federal legislation enacted from 1968 to 1972 established comprehensive Medicare, the national health insurance system; subsequent legislation put even more restrictions on private health care. See Canada Health Act, 1984, available at www.hc-sc.gc.ca/medicare/Canada%20Health%20Act.htm.

3. John R. Graham and Nadeem Esmail, "The BC Government Is Eroding Patients' and Physicians' Rights," Fraser Institute (December 10, 2003), and interview with the authors; an abridged version appeared in *The Province*, Vancouver, British Columbia (December 10, 2003).

4. In one case, a public hospital sold MRI scans after hours for use by veterinarians on pets. This proved to be controversial, however, and a public outcry forced the program's cancellation. See Jeff Harder, "Hospitals Profit from Pets," *CNEWS,* December 18, 1998; Thomas Walkom, "No Pets Ahead of People. Health Ministry Says Leadership Candidate Eves Was Mistaken about MRI Availability," *Toronto Star*, January 11, 2002. There is, however, a health private market for pet treatments. See Robert Scalia, "Health Care: No Waiting Lists," *Montreal Gazette*, November 30, 2003; Frank Calleja, "Royal Treatment for a Sick Rover. $5M Animal Hospital to Treat Cancer. Oakville Facility to Be State of the Art," *Toronto Star,* September 25, 2003.

5. The draft EU constitution states, "Everyone has the right of access to preventive health care and the right to benefit from medical treatment under the conditions established by national laws and practices." European Union draft constitution, Part II (The Charter of Fundamental Rights of the Union), Title IV, Article II-35 on Health Care. Available at http://europa.eu.int/eur-lex/en/treaties/dat/C2003169en.002201.htm.

6. Long before the advances of modern medicine, Enoch Powell, former British minister of health, argued that waiting lines are inevitable under the NHS, regardless of the resources devoted to health care. See Enoch Powell, *Medicine and Politics, 1975 and After* (New York: Pitman, 1976). For a discussion of British hospital rationing, see John C. Goodman, *National Health Care in Great Britain: Lessons for the U.S.A.* (Dallas: Fisher Institute, 1980), ch. 6.

7. "Waiting List Figures, November 2001," UK Department of Health, Statistical Press Release, January 11, 2002.

8. Nadeem Esmail and Michael Walker, "Waiting Your Turn: Hospital Waiting Lists in Canada, 13th Edition," *Fraser Institute, Critical Issues Bulletin,* October 2003.

9. Michael Hoel and Erik Magnus Saether, "Private Health Care as a Supplement to a Public Health System with Waiting Time for Treatment," Frisch Center for Economic Research, Oslo, Norway, 2000.

10. "Purchasing for Your Health 1996/97," New Zealand Ministry of Health, March 1998.

11. Hospital admissions as a percent of the total population average 16.01 percent for all OECD countries. The figures are 16.0 percent for the United Kingdom, 13.8 percent for New Zealand and 11.0 percent for Canada. See Gerald F. Anderson and Jean-Pierre Poullier, "Health Spending, Access, and Outcomes: Trends in Industrialized Countries," *Health Affairs* 18, no. 3 (1999): 178–92

12. See Hoel and Saether, "Private Health Care as a Supplement."

13. Esmail and Walker, "Waiting Your Turn."

14. "Purchasing for Your Health 1996/97," Figures 5.13 and 5.14.

15. "Purchasing for Your Health 1996/97," Figures 5.13 and 5.14.

16. Michael White and John Carvel, "Private Ops Offer to Cut NHS Queue," *The Guardian*, December 6, 2001.

17. Matthew Young and Eamonn Butler, "The Million-Year Wait," Adam Smith Institute, 2002.

18. Esmail and Walker, "Waiting Your Turn."

19. Hospital Inpatient Statistics, NHS Trust Based: "Green Book" Index for 2001/02 Department of Health, 2002.

20. Hospital Inpatient Statistics, NHS Trust Based: "Green Book" Index for 2001/02 Department of Health, 2002.

21. Karol Sikora and Nick Bosanquet, "Cancer Care in the United Kingdom: New Solutions Are Needed," *British Medical Journal* (November 1, 2003): 1044–46.

22. Sir John Bourn (Comptroller and Auditor General), "Inappropriate Adjustments to NHS Waiting Lists," UK National Audit Office, December 19, 2001.

23. Andrew Smithers, "The Real Problem Budget Must Aim to Solve," *Evening Standard*, April 10, 2002.

24. Anthony Browne, "Cash-Strapped NHS Hospitals Chase Private Patient 'Bonanza'," *The Observer*, December 16, 2001. Also see Browne, "Deadly Rise in Wait for Cancer Care," *The Observer*, March 3, 2002; and Browne, "How Thousands of Cancer Patients and Doctors Have Been Betrayed," *The Observer*, March 3, 2002.

25. Similar results are likely true of other cancers as well. See Noelle O'Rourke and R. Edwards, "Lung Cancer Treatment Waiting Times and Tumour Growth," *Clinical Oncology* (Royal College of Radiologists) 12, no. 3 (June 2000): 141–44, cited in Kirsty Scott, "Treatment Delays Are Killing Cancer Patients," *The Guardian*, July 1, 2000.

26. Anthony Browne and Matthew Young, "NHS reform: Towards Consensus?" *A Partnership for Better Health Report,* Adam Smith Institute, 2002. Approximately 130,000 people in England die of heart disease each year. However, the NHS estimates that only 500 cardiac patients die annually while waiting for care. See Linda

Beecham, "Health Secretary Will Target Heart Disease," *British Medical Journal* (October 23, 1999); "500 Heart Patients Die on Waiting Lists," *BBC News,* June 3, 1999.

27. Audit Commission, "Waiting for Elective Admission: Review of National Findings," in *Health: Acute Hospital Portfolio* (London: Audit Commission, June 2003).

28. "Canadian Health Care—A System in Collapse," Fraser Institute, *Backgrounder*, 1999.

29. Paul McDonald et al., "Waiting Lists and Waiting Times for Health Care in Canada: More Management! More Money?" Health Canada, Summary Report, July 1998.

30. This figure also includes coronary patients previously treated in Britain who suffered a subsequent heart attack while in Europe.

31. Celia Hall, "Thousand NHS Patients Treated Abroad," *The Daily Telegraph*, August 21, 2001.

32. "More People Will Pay for Healthcare," *BBC News,* May 30, 2001.

33. See Panos Kanavos, Martin McKee and Tessa Richards, "Cross-Border Health Care in Europe," *British Medical Journal* (May 1, 1999):1157–58.

34. Jan Ove Nesse, "Norwegian Patients in EU Hospitals: The Medical Treatment Abroad Project," Norwegian Insurance Administration, December 2001, 3.

35. Kanavos, McKee and Richards, "Cross-Border Health Care in Europe."

36. One British shadow health secretary, Liam Fox, has advocated allowing patients to shop for private care with NHS cash in circumstances when the NHS cannot provide timely care. See David Charter, "Fox Plan Would Allow Patients to Shop Around," *The Times* (London), October 8, 2002; Alice Miles, "A Bold Health Policy to Make Blair Sick with Envy," *The Times* (London), October 8, 2002.

37. Peter Landers, "Longer Dialysis Offers New Hope But Poses Dilemma," *Wall Street Journal,* October 2, 2002.

38. The HeartMate is a small implantable blood pump made out of titanium. The therapy is called Left Ventricular Assist System and is used to support patients with end-stage heart failure who are not eligible for heart transplantation. Theresa Agovino, "Price of Heart Device May Mean Rationing," Associated Press, *Miami Herald,* September 1, 2003.

39. Antonio Regalado, "To Sell Pricey Drug, Lilly Fuels a Debate over Rationing," *Wall Street Journal,* September 18, 2003.

40. Gina Kolata, "50 and Ready for a Colonoscopy? Doctors Say There Is Often a Wait," *New York Times*, December 8, 2003.

41. One of the best new tools for detecting cancer is the Positron Emission Tomography (PET) scanner, which uses radioactive drugs to detect tumors.

42. Results of July 2002 Society of Critical Care Medicine poll. Reported in Regalado, "To Sell Pricey Drug, Lilly Fuels a Debate over Rationing."

Chapter Two

Equality

MYTH NO. 2: IN COUNTRIES WITH SINGLE-PAYER NATIONAL HEALTH CARE SYSTEMS, ALL PEOPLE HAVE EQUAL ACCESS TO HEALTH CARE

One of the most surprising features of single-payer care systems is the enormous amount of rhetoric devoted to the notion of equality and the importance of achieving it, especially in relation to the tiny amount of progress that appears to have been made. "Only a single comprehensive program, covering rich and poor alike, can end disparities based on race, ethnicity, social class, and geographic region, . . ." claims the U.S. Physicians' Working Group for Single-Payer National Health Insurance.[1]

Similar sentiments were expressed when the British NHS was established in 1948. Aneurin Bevan, father of the NHS, declared that "everyone should be treated alike in the matter of medical care."[2] The Beveridge Report, the blueprint for the NHS, promised "a health service providing full preventive and curative treatment of every kind for every citizen without exceptions."[3] The *British Medical Journal* predicted in 1942 that the NHS would be "a 100 percent service for 100 percent of the population."[4] The goal of the NHS founders was to eliminate inequalities in health care based on age, sex, occupation, geographical location and—most importantly—income and social class. As Bevan put it, "the essence of a satisfactory health service is that rich and poor are treated alike, that poverty is not a disability and wealth is not advantaged."[5] Similar statements have been made by politicians in virtually every country that has established a national health insurance program. Yet, such rhetoric rarely corresponds with the facts.

27

INEQUALITY IN BRITAIN

Britain's ministers of health have long assured Britons that they were leaving no stone unturned in a relentless quest to root out and eliminate inequalities in health care. But more than thirty years into the program (in the 1980s), an official task force (the Black Report) found little evidence that access to health care was any more equal than when the NHS was started.[6] Almost twenty years later, a second task force (the Acheson Report) found evidence that access had become less equal in the years between the two studies.[7]

Across a range of indices, NHS performance figures have consistently shown widening gaps between the best-performing and worst-performing hospitals and health authorities, as well as vastly different survival rates for different types of illness, depending on where patients live. The problem of unequal access is so well known in Britain that the press refers to the NHS as a "postcode lottery" in which a person's chances for timely, high-quality treatment depend on the neighborhood or "postcode" in which he or she lives.[8]

"Generally speaking, the poorer you are and the more socially deprived your area, the worse your care and access is likely to be," says *The Guardian,* a staunch defender of socialized medicine.[9] Scholarly studies of the issue have come to similar conclusions. For example, a study by the Joseph Rowntree Research Trust published in 2000 found discrepancies among areas for all causes of death:[10]

- Nonelderly Britons living in areas with the worst-performing hospitals were 42 percent more likely to die on any given day than the average for Britain as a whole.
- The nonelderly population living in regions with the best-performing hospitals were 24 percent less likely to die than the average for Britain as a whole.
- Overall, the study found that if health care inequity were merely decreased to 1983 levels, some 7,500 premature deaths among people younger than sixty-five could be avoided each year.

Other researchers reinforce these conclusions:

- One study found that if the proportion of cancer-related illnesses and deaths were the same in Britain's lowest socioeconomic groups as in the most affluent, there would be 16,600 fewer deaths from cancer each year.[11]
- The British Heart Foundation (BHF) found that the premature death rate for working-class men is 58 percent higher than non-working-class men;[12] the BHF estimates that more than 5,000 working-class men under the age of sixty-five die of coronary heart disease each year in Britain because of variations in health care access for different socioeconomic groups.[13]

TABLE 2-1

Good Hospital Guide:
How London Hospitals Compare

	Hospital	Mortality Index[1]	Drs per 100 Beds	Nurses per 100 Beds
1	Univ. Coll. London Hosp*	68	63	180
2	Bart's and the London*	70	53	129
3	Royal Free Hampstead*	79	48	131
4	Chelsea/Westm'ter H'care*	82	64	169
5	Guy's and St. Thomas's*	82	59	161
6	North West London Hosps	85	53	129
7	Hammersmith Hospitals	88	41	126
8	North Middlesex Hospital	88	49	119
9	Whittington Hospital*	90	43	150
10	St. George's Healthcare	91	49	123
11	St. Mary's Hospital*	91	59	132
12	Homerton Hospital*	92	33	116
13	King's College Hospital*	95	54	136
14	Bromley Hospitals	97	38	95
15	Kingston Hospital	101	57	169
16	Epsom and St. Helier	102	38	108
17	Queen Mary's Sidcup	103	37	109
18	Ealing Hospitals	103	42	122
19	Forest Healthcare	106	25	86
20	Lewisham Hospital*	106	37	131
21	Barnet and Chase Farm	106	43	150
22	Redbridge Healthcare	108	19	75
23	Mayday Healthcare	108	32	93
24	West Middox Univ Hospital	109	45	144
25	Newham Healthcare*	109	29	70
26	Hillingdon Hospital	111	33	108
27	Havering Hospitals	112	36	107
28	Greenwich Healthcare	112	17	131

[1] The mortality index is adjusted for severity of cases and is ranked from low to high. Average index for London region: 96.

* Indicates Inner London boroughs (average mortality index: Inner London 85; Outer London 102).

Source: Dr. Foster, *The Good Hospital Guide* (London: Dr. Foster, Ltd., January 2001).

The disparity between rich and poor areas in Britain was confirmed by *The Good Hospital Guide*, which graded every hospital in Britain according to a mortality index.[14] The index was calculated so that a hospital with a survival rate that matched exactly the national average scored 100 points. Hospitals with a lower survival rate than the national average scored above 100, while those with a higher survival rate scored below. The disparity was especially striking among London hospitals. Table 2.1 shows the following:

- The hospitals with the best performance, University College London Hospital, Royal Free Hampstead and Chelsea/Westminster, are located in the center of London, in or near the wealthiest sectors of the city.
- The hospitals with the worst performance, Greenwich, Havering, Redbridge and Newham, are located in east London, the most economically depressed area of the city.
- In addition, there are nearly four times as many doctors per 100 patients at Chelsea/Westminster (64) as in Greenwich (17).

Overall, the study found a correlation between a region's socioeconomic conditions, the quality of its health care services and the survival rates of its patients. Generally, hospitals in richer areas are more likely to have more staff per hospital bed, and their patients are more likely to survive treatment than patients in poor areas.

There are also differences in health outcomes. For example, a man with prostate cancer in Bexley and Greenwich in southeast London has a 34 percent chance of surviving for five years, while a man in the Kensington/Westminster area has a 60 percent chance.[15]

INEQUALITY IN CANADA

Canadian officials also put a high premium on equality of access to medical care. In 1999, for instance, Health Minister Allan Rock stated, "Equal access regardless of financial means will continue to be a cornerstone of our system."[16] How well have the Canadians done? A series of studies from the University of British Columbia in the 1990s consistently found widespread inequality in the provision of care among British Columbia's twenty or so health regions. These studies are unique because researchers identified patients by the region in which they live rather than the region where they received care. This allowed investigators to identify inequities in the amount of care received by residents of each region, including those patients forced to travel hundreds of miles (from one region to another) for treatment.[17]

For example, take the amount spent on the services of physician specialists for Vancouver, the largest city, with a population of almost two million, and Peace River, a rural area of about 60,000. As table 2.2 shows,[18]

TABLE 2-2

Services of All Specialists for Residents of Two Areas in Canada
(Spending per person)[1]

	Vancouver[2]	Peace River[3]
Child, Age 0-4:		
Male	$727.4	$242.5
Female	639.0	202.5
Child, Age 5-9:		
Male	421.9	114.3
Female	361.4	105.2
Adult, Age 40-59:		
Male	579.4	163.3
Female	773.1	271.7
Adult, Age 70-79:		
Male	1,302.0	452.4
Female	1,044.1	484.8
All ages:		
All specialists	609.5	231.6
Internists	50.5	11.6
OB/GYNs	18.1	6.5
Psychiatrists	31.8	1.5

[1] Includes all physicians' fees for services rendered to residents living in the areas indicated, regardless of the area in which the service was received. Spending figures are age/sex standardized and are expressed in Canadian dollars.

[2] Greater Vancouver Regional Hospital District, British Columbia.

[3] Peace River Regional Hospital District, British Columbia.

Source: Arminée Kazanjian et al., "Fee Practice Medical Expenditures per Capita and Full-Time-Equivalent Physicians in British Columbia, 1993-94," University of British Columbia, 1995.

- Residents of Vancouver received almost three times more specialist services per person than residents of Peace River, and this inequality held for groups with comparable health needs, males and females, and across all age groups.
- The differences were even more striking for certain specialties, with a five-to-one difference in the services of internists and a thirty-one-to-one difference in the services of psychiatrists.

One might suppose that a higher level of GP services would offset the lower level of specialist services in Peace River. As figure 2.1 shows, that was not the case. Vancouver residents also enjoyed about 60 percent more GP services.

FIGURE 2-1

Amounts Spent on Physician Services for Residents of Two Canadian Hospital Districts[1]

(Per capita spending)

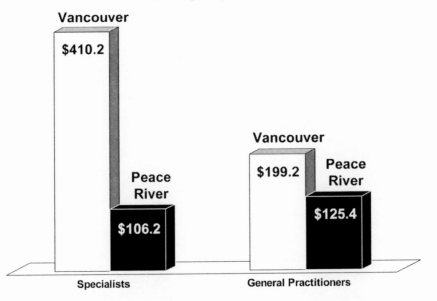

[1] Figures are expressed in Canadian dollars and are age/sex standardized.

Source: Arminée Kazanjian et al., "Fee Practice Medical Expenditures Per Capita and Full-Time-Equivalent Physicians in British Columbia, 1993-94," University of British Columbia, 1995.

In general, spending on medical services varied widely by region throughout British Columbia. As table 2.3 shows,[19]

- Spending on specialist services in Vancouver was almost four times higher than spending on specialists in rural Cariboo.
- Per capita spending on all services was almost three times as high in Vancouver ($609) as in Peace River ($231).
- Differences between the lowest- and highest-spending regions in British Columbia were especially striking in certain specialties—a fourfold difference in spending on internal medicine, a thirty-one-fold difference in spending on psychiatric services and a fourfold difference in spending on obstetrics-gynecology (OB/GYN).

TABLE 2-3

Spending per Person on Physician Services By Hospital Districts in British Columbia[1]

Hospital Districts	Total Spending	Specialists	OB/GYN	Psychi-atrists	Internists
Urban districts:					
Vancouver	$609.5	$410.2	$18.1	$31.8	$50.5
Victoria	379.5	242.4	8.9	13.3	28.0
Average	494.5				
Selected Rural Districts:					
North Okanagan	290.8	153.8	7.9	4.1	16.3
Cariboo	265.3	125.5	7.8	2.5	17.0
Upper Fraser Valley	309.2	172.3	8.6	6.0	19.4
Central Kootenay	301.9	157.5	7.0	1.8	22.3
East Kootenay	267.0	119.8	3.5	0.8	10.2
South Okanagan	324.0	196.8	10.3	9.4	32.0
Simon Fraser	415.7	281.4	8.5	9.3	33.4
Peace River	231.6	106.2	6.5	1.0	11.6
Skeena-Queen	273.2	149.4	6.3	1.0	19.0
Burnaby	282.6	169.2	7.5	16.5	23.2
North Shore	338.6	206.7	7.6	13.2	27.9
Central Fraser Valley	278.8	151.9	8.4	7.1	20.5
Richmond	301.1	182.4	7.9	13.3	28.0
Average	289.5				

[1] Based on fees paid to physicians for rendering services to patients living in the areas indicated, regardless of the area in which the service was performed. All figures are age-sex standardized and expressed in Canadian dollars.

Source: Arminée Kazanjian et al., "Fee Practice Medical Expenditures per capita and Full-Time-Equivalent Physicians in British Columbia, 1993-94," University of British Columbia, 1995.

These results are now a decade old, and the study has not been repeated. However, as we shall see below, the same researchers have continued to track the supply of resources on a region-by-region basis, and inequalities of supply have continued through time and in some cases gotten worse.

In most countries with waiting lists for care, the poor wait longer than the wealthy and powerful. For example, a survey of Ontario physicians found more than 80 percent of physicians, including 90 percent of cardiac surgeons, 81 percent of internists and 60 percent of family physicians had been personally involved in managing a patient who had received preferential access on the basis of factors other than medical need. When asked about those patients most likely to receive preferential treatment, physicians reported that 93 percent had personal ties to the treating physician, 85 percent were high-profile public figures and 83 percent were politicians.[20]

Other studies have reached similar conclusions. One study found that the wealthy and powerful have significantly greater access to medical specialists than the less-well-connected poor.[21] A University of Toronto study finds that high-profile patients enjoy more frequent services, shorter waiting times and greater choice in specialists.[22]

These findings are supported by anecdotal evidence. In recent years, the Canadian media has reported numerous examples of wealthy and prominent patients "jumping the queue" for quicker treatment, while ordinary citizens languish.[23] For example, Canada's health minister, Allan Rock, underwent a successful surgery after he was diagnosed with prostate cancer in January 2001. Rock was sharply criticized by other Canadian prostate cancer patients who waited much longer for treatment, often more than a year between diagnosis and surgery.[24] The president of the Canadian Medical Association, Dr. Victor Dirnfeld, suggested in 1998 that the Canadian system is in fact a two-tiered system, and said that he knew of seven prominent political figures in British Columbia and Ontario who received special treatment. "Instead of waiting three months for an MRI," he said, "they will have it done in three or four days."[25]

Despite the removal of financial barriers, Canadians apparently do not have equal access to health care. Access is influenced by education and income as well as political influence.[26]

ACCESS IN THE UNITED STATES

There are also disparities in access to health care in the United States. The latest count shows that 43.6 million Americans, approximately 15.2 percent of the U.S. population, lack private health insurance and are not enrolled in public health programs.[27] Studies show that the uninsured consume about 50 percent less health care than those with insurance, other things being equal.[28]

Many of the uninsured are uninsured by choice, which implies that they have no problem paying for the care they need, they are getting free care, or they are relatively healthy and do not see a need for insurance. For example, about one-third of the uninsured qualify for government coverage through S-CHIP (for low-income children)[29] and Medicaid (for low-income families), but have not enrolled. Roughly one-third live in households with incomes above $50,000 and apparently can afford health insurance even though they choose not to purchase it. In fact, within the last seven to eight years, virtually all of the increase in the uninsured has been among families with incomes in excess of $50,000 and more than half of those earn $80,000 a year or more. Of those who become uninsured at any point in time, Census Bureau data show that about three-quarters (74.7 percent) obtain insurance within one year, while only 2.5 percent remain uninsured for more than three years.[30]

For decades, the socialist press in Europe has repeated the canard that poor people in the United States get no care because they cannot afford it. Nothing could be further from the truth. Almost all of the elderly (including the low-income elderly) are enrolled in Medicare, through which they are entitled to virtually all the U.S. health care system has to offer (with some exceptions noted in chapter 1).[31] Furthermore, Medicaid, the federal-state program for the poor, now spends more than Medicare even though it covers roughly the same number of people; and those who enroll in Medicaid and seek care use services at rates comparable to those with private insurance.[32] The Veterans Administration provides yet another safety net. And, every state has a system of public hospitals and clinics that provide medical services to the indigent.

Despite the European notion that the poor and the uninsured are turned away at the hospital admitting room door, federal law requires emergency rooms to take all comers, regardless of ability to pay.[33] State and federal laws also require many hospitals to provide charity care, and federal and state matching funds are available to institutions that provide a disproportionate share of care to Medicaid patients and the uninsured. Through these multiple channels, the poor often have access to the most advanced technology and therapies.

A study by the Texas Comptroller of Public Accounts found that public and private organizations in Texas spend, on the average, approximately $1,000 per year on care for each uninsured Texan.[34] This is equivalent to $4,000 for a family of four, enough to buy private health insurance in many Texas cities. Another study from the Urban Institute in Washington, D.C., found that the United States spends $34.5 billion on free health care for the uninsured, or about $820 per person each year.[35] If the value of uncompensated physicians' time is included, the amount probably exceeds $1,000 per uninsured individual. Further, evidence from Texas indicates that free care for the uninsured and spending on Medicaid tend to be substitutes for each other. That is, those health regions that spend more through Medicaid, spend less on free care and vice versa.[36]

To see what this means on the local level, consider Parkland Hospital in Dallas, a primary source of care for the indigent as well as those covered by Medicaid. Although many studies suggest that being uninsured results in less health care, this conclusion would not be at all obvious to an observer sitting in Parkland's emergency room. Uninsured patients and Medicaid patients pass through the same emergency room door; they see the same doctors; they receive the same treatments; and if required, they are admitted to hospital rooms on the same floors.

The only people who seem to care very much about who is insured or uninsured at Parkland are the hospital staff (presumably because that affects how they get paid). For that reason, employees work their way through the emergency room waiting area in an attempt to enroll all eligible patients in Medicaid (most of the time they fail). With the same goal in mind, employees also go room to room to visit those who are admitted (their success rate is much higher).

Interestingly, eligible patients in Texas can enroll in Medicaid and have the state pay their medical bills three months after the fact. So if there is any reason for a patient to enroll, clearly there is no need for haste.

At Children's Medical Center, next door to Parkland, a similar exercise takes place. Children on Medicaid, children on S-CHIP (for low-income families who do not qualify for Medicaid), and uninsured children all come through the same emergency room door. Again, they all see the same doctors and receive the same treatments. Again, it is only the hospital that seems to care whether anybody is insured and by whom.

The experiences of these two hospitals illustrates that the uninsured in America are often not uninsured in any real sense of the term. Many of them get their care in hospital emergency rooms, just as many Canadians and Britons do. They do not pay for the care they receive and often are not even sent a bill, just like in London or Toronto. It is only on paper and in statistics examined by academic researchers that the patients in London and Toronto are classified as "insured," while U.S. patients are "uninsured." The difference appears to be one of form, not of substance.

Europeans who have grown up on a steady diet of anti-American-health-care propaganda would probably be surprised to learn how much Americans actually spend on health care for low-income families. Each year, Medicaid costs U.S. taxpayers almost $1,000 for every man, woman and child in the country, or $4,000 for a family of four.[37] Free care for the uninsured costs another $4,000. And if taxpayer support for the low- and moderate-income elderly are included, the average family of four is probably spending $10,000 or more on other people's health care. Indeed, most taxpayers with private insurance are paying far more in taxes to fund health insurance for other people than they pay for private health insurance for themselves and their own families.

Low-income beneficiaries on Medicaid probably have more access to better health care than low-income citizens in any other country. According to a recent study by Health Services Research,[38]

- Low-income persons in the United States without job-related health insurance spend only about fifty dollars per year more out of pocket for health services than those with employer-provided health benefits.
- On the average, they make 2.4 visits to physicians each year, compared to 3.4 visits for persons with employer-provided insurance coverage.
- However, when seriously ill, uninsured low- and moderate-income Americans receive about the same level of treatment and services as those with employment-based coverage, and their out-of-pocket costs are about the same.

This suggests that the health care safety net in the United States is actually more reliable than many people think. About 3 percent of the U.S. population is uninsured for six months or longer. By contrast, one study found that about 5 percent of British Columbians are not registered for the provincial health insurance program and are therefore uninsured.[39] Almost all of these uninsured Canadians are poor. Like the Medicaid-eligible uninsured in the United States, they need only register to become formally insured.

COMPARING THE UNITED STATES WITH OTHER COUNTRIES

There are inequalities in access to health care in every country. Low-income people in almost every country see physicians less often, spend less time with them, enter the hospital less often and spend less time there, especially when the use of medical services is weighted by the incidence of illness. As we shall see, this is only partly due to barriers people face in obtaining care. However, in the United States, patients say the main barrier is financial; in countries that have presumably removed financial barriers to care, there are other barriers.

In an international opinion survey sponsored by the Commonwealth Fund, 21 percent of Americans said they had serious problems paying for health care compared to only 11 percent in Canada.[40] Roughly the same proportion of Americans (17 percent) and Canadians (16 percent) had experienced difficulty seeing a medical specialist when needed. In the United States, cost was most frequently cited as the major obstacle, while waiting times and physician shortages were the main barriers in Britain and Canada.[41] In fact, among patients who describe themselves as in "fair" or "poor" health, the percent who experience long waits to see specialists is twice as high in Canada as in the United States.[42] (See the discussion in chapter 6.)

Another survey queried those who rated their health as "fair" or "poor" about the "biggest problem with their respective health care system." While only 13 percent of Canadians complained about the high cost of health care, 16 percent cited inadequate government funding, 27 percent complained about waiting times, and 54 percent cited a shortage of health care professionals and hospital beds.[43] By contrast, 48 percent of Americans complained about the high cost of health care. Only 1 percent, 3 percent and 5 percent of Americans (respectively) complained about inadequate government funding, waiting lines or a shortage of health care professionals and hospital beds.[44]

NOTES

1. Marcia Angell et al., Physicians' Working Group on Single-Payer National Health Insurance, "Proposal for Health Care Reform," Presentation to the Congressional Black Caucus and the Congressional Progressive Caucus, May 1, 2001.

2. Quoted in Economic Models, Ltd., *The British Health Care System* (Chicago: American Medical Association, 1976), 33.

3. Quoted in Harry Swartz, "The Infirmity of British Medicine," in *The Future That Doesn't Work: Social Democracy's Failures in Britain*, Emmett Tyrrell Jr., ed. (New York: Doubleday, 1977), 24.

4. *British Medical Journal* (December 12, 1942): 700.

5. Aneurin Bevan, *In Place of Fear* (London: Heinemann, 1952), 76.

6. *Inequalities in Health*, Black Report (London: UK Department of Health and Social Security, 1980).

7. *Independent Inquiry into Inequalities in Health*, Acheson Report (London: Stationery Office, 1998). See also "Geographic Variations in Health," UK Office for National Statistics, Decennial Supplement 16, 2001.

8. See, for example, "Postcode Lottery in Social Services," *BBC News*, October 13, 2000; "New Health Tables Reveal Postcode Lottery,"*Ananova.com*, July 14, 2000; and "'Regional Lottery' of Hospital Waiting Times," *Ananova.com*, August 31, 2000.

9. Patrick Butler, "Q&A: Postcode Lottery," *The Guardian* (Manchester), November 8, 2000.

10. Dr. Richard Mitchell and Dr. Mary Shaw, "Reducing Health Inequalities in Britain," Joseph Rowntree Foundation, September 2000.

11. "Cancer Trends in England and Wales, 1950–1999," *Health Statistics Quarterly*, no. 8 (Winter 2000), 18.

12. "Coronary Heart Disease Statistics," British Heart Foundation, Statistics Database, 1998.

13. Sir Charles George, "Coronary Heart Disease Statistics," British Heart Foundation, 1999.

14. Dr. Foster, *The Good Hospital Guide* (London: Dr. Foster, Ltd. January 14, 2001).

15. Data based on clinical indicators published by the British Department of Health. See Sebastian O'Kelly, "Consumer: Lottery of Life and Death," *The Guardian* (Manchester), October 1, 1998.

16. News release, "Minister Rock Announces Funding for Community Health and Research Initiatives in Alberta," Regional News Release, 1999–1992, *Health Canada* (July 12, 1999).

17. Arminée Kazanjian et al., "Fee Practice Medical Expenditures per Capita and Full-Time Equivalent Physicians in British Columbia, 1993–1994," University of British Columbia, Centre for Health Services and Policy Research, 1995.

18. A new series of studies from British Columbia tracks full-time equivalent (FTE) physicians by region. These studies show far more physicians per capita in urban areas than in rural ones. Arminée Kazanjian, Alice Chen, Laura Wood and Patrick Wong Fung, "Doctors & Patients: Supply, Use and Payments in British Columbia, 1998–1999," Part I—Physician FTEs and Distribution in B.C., Centre for Health Services and Policy Research, University of British Columbia, June 2001. The "Doctors & Patients" reports are an updated version of the HHRU series of reports formerly titled "Fee Practice Medical Services Expenditures per Capita and Full-Time-Equivalent (FTE) Physicians."

19. Arminée Kazanjian et al., "Fee Practice Medical Expenditures."

20. A. S. Basinski and C. D. Naylor, "A Survey of Provider Experiences and Perceptions of Preferential Access to Cardiovascular Care in Ontario, Canada," *Annals of Internal Medicine* 129, no. 7, 1998.

21. David A. Alter et al., "Effects of Socioeconomic Status on Access to Invasive Cardiac Procedures and on Mortality after Acute Myocardial Infarction," *New England Journal of Medicine* 341, no. 18 (October 28, 1999): 1359–67.

22. Sheryl Dunlop, Peter C. Coyte and Warren McIsaac, "Socio-Economic Status and the Utilisation of Physicians' Services: Results from the Canadian National Population Health Survey," *Social Science and Medicine* 51, no. 1 (July 2000): 1–11.

23. "Well-Connected Patients Skip to Head of Line," *Ottawa Citizen*, October 1, 1998; "Province to Pay Costs of MRI Scans since '93," *Calgary Herald*, April 10, 2001; Maria Bohuslawsky, "Politicians Jump Medicare Queue," *Ottawa Citizen*, June 6, 1998; and "Queue-Jumping Privatizes Medicare," *Toronto Star Health Reporter*, March 31, 1999.

24. Jake Rupert, "Man Protests Rock's Speedy Surgery," *Ottawa Citizen*, February 17, 2001.

25. Bohuslawsky, "Politicians Jump Medicare Queue."

26. Lisa Priest, "Study Shows Rich More Likely to See Medical Specialist," *Toronto Globe and Mail*, April 25, 2000.

27. Robert J. Mills and Shailesh Bhandari, "Health Insurance Coverage in the United States: 2002," *Current Population Reports*, U.S. Census Bureau, U.S. Department of Commerce, September 2003, 60–223; and U.S. Census Bureau, "Health Insurance Coverage—1993," Statistical Brief, SB/94–28, October 1994.

28. M. Susan Marquis and Stephen H. Long, "The Uninsured Access Gap: Narrowing the Estimates," *Inquiry* 31 (Winter 1994/95): 405–14. Marquis and Long found that uninsured adults have about 60 percent as many physician visits and 70 percent as many inpatient hospital days as they would if they were covered by insurance. See also M. Susan Marquis and Stephen H. Long, "The Uninsured 'Access Gap' and the Cost of Universal Coverage," *Health Affairs* (Spring [II] 1994): 211–20.

29. The State Children's Health Insurance Program (S-CHIP) was created by the Balanced Budget Act of 1997 (BBA). It is a federal-state program designed to insure children in families with incomes too high for Medicaid but too low to be able to afford private health insurance.

30. Devon M. Herrick, "Uninsured by Choice: Update," Brief Analysis No. 460, National Center for Policy Analysis, October 7, 2003, available at www.ncpa.org/pub/ba/ba460.

31. Low-income seniors are also covered by Medicaid, the program that provides health care to the indigent.

32. M. Susan Marquis and Stephen H. Long, "Reconsidering the Effect of Medicaid on Health Care Services Use," *Health Services Research* 30, no. 6 (February 1996): 792–808.

33. The law that requires hospitals with emergency rooms to treat (or stabilize before transferring) emergency patients is the Consolidated Omnibus Budget Reconciliation Act (COBRA) of 1985. See Joseph P. Wood, "Emergency Physicians' Obligations to Managed Care Patients under COBRA," *Academic Emergency Medicine* 3, no. 8 (August 1996): 794–800.

34. Naomi Lopez Bauman and Devon M. Herrick, "Uninsured in the Lone Star State," National Center for Policy Analysis, Brief Analysis No. 335, August 29, 2000.

35. Jack Hadley and John Holahan, "How Much Medical Care Do the Uninsured Use, and Who Pays for It?" *Health Affairs* (February 12, 2003) (Web exclusive).

36. Sen. Chris Harris (Chairman) et al., "Texas Blue Ribbon Task Force on the Uninsured: Report to the 77th Legislature," State of Texas, February 2001.

37. Michael Bond, John C. Goodman, Ronald Lindsey, and Richard Teske, "Reforming Medicaid," National Center for Policy Analysis, Policy Report No. 257, February 2003.

38. Richard W. Johnson and Stephen Crystal, "Uninsured Status and Out-of-Pocket Costs at Midlife," *Health Services Research* 35, no. 5, Part I (December 2000): 911–32.

39. Two provinces, Alberta and British Columbia, charge premiums, and people who do not pay them are technically uninsured. See Edmund F. Haislmaier, "Problems in Paradise: Canadians Complain about their Health Care System," *Back-*

grounder, no. 883, Heritage Foundation, February 19, 1992. It was reported that at one Vancouver hospital, nearly 10 percent of the patients in the emergency room were uninsured. See Linda Gorman, "Paying Twice for Government Health Care," Independence Institute, August 30, 2001.

40. Cathy Schoen, Robert J. Blendon, Catherine M. DesRoches, and Robin Osborn, "Comparison of Health Care System Views and Experiences in Five Nations, 2001," Issue Brief, Commonwealth Fund, May 2002, available at www.cmwf.org/programs/international/schoen_fivenation_ib_542.pdf.

41. Schoen et al., "Comparison of Health Care System Views."

42. See Robert J. Blendon, Cathy Schoen, Catherine M. DesRoches, Robin Osborn, et al., "Inequities in Health Care: A Five Country Survey," *Health Affairs* 21, no. 3 (May/June 2002): 182–91; and Robert J. Blendon et al., "Common Concerns Amid Diverse Systems: Health Care Experiences in Five Countries," *Health Affairs* 22, no. 3 (May/June 2003): 106–21.

43. Blendon et al., "Common Concerns Amid Diverse Systems," Exhibit 2.

44. Blendon et al., "Common Concerns Amid Diverse Systems."

Chapter Three

Needs

MYTH NO. 3: COUNTRIES WITH SINGLE-PAYER NATIONAL HEALTH INSURANCE MAKE HEALTH CARE AVAILABLE ON THE BASIS OF NEED RATHER THAN ABILITY TO PAY

"The United States alone treats health care as a commodity distributed according to the ability to pay, rather than as a social service to be distributed according to medical need," claims Physicians for Single-Payer National Health Insurance. This is an article of faith among supporters of socialized medicine. Indeed, Aneurin Bevan, father of the British NHS, resigned from the Labor government in 1951 when a small charge was instituted for dental services and prescription drugs. As a matter of principle, he explained, health care should be free to the patient.

But is it really true that single-payer systems make care available on the basis of need alone? Precisely because of rationing, inefficiencies and quality problems, patients in single-payer countries often spend their own money on health care when they are given an opportunity to do so. In fact, private-sector health care is the fastest-growing part of the health care system in many of these countries. For example:

- In the first six years of the 1990s, private medical spending in Sweden rose 62 percent, to slightly less than 16 percent of total medical expenditure.[1]
- Over the same period, private medical spending in Ireland rose to 25 percent of the health care market.
- In Britain, 13 percent of the population has private health insurance, to cover services they presumably are entitled to for free under the NHS, and

private sector spending makes up 15 percent of the country's total health care spending.[2]

- In Canada, the share of privately funded health care spending rose from 24 percent in 1983 to an estimated 30.3 percent in 1998.[3]
- In Australia, private health insurance coverage has risen from around 31 percent in 1998 to almost 45 percent of the population by March 2002.[4]
- In New Zealand, 35 percent of the population has private health insurance (again, to cover services theoretically provided for free by the state), and private sector spending is about 10 percent of total health care spending.[5]

PRIVATE HEALTH CARE IN BRITAIN

Under the NHS, people have always had the right to pay for private treatment.[6] And despite British claims that health care is a right that is not conditioned on the ability to pay, last year an estimated 100,000 patients elected to pay for private surgery rather than wait for "free" care.[7] These patients went to one of Britain's 300 private hospitals, which account for an increasingly large share of total health care services, including 20 percent of all nonemergency heart surgery and 30 percent of all hip replacements.[8]

Altogether, almost seven million people are covered by private health insurance and they account for two-thirds of all patients in private hospitals. The existence of a large private health care industry suggests that many Britons are willing to spend more on their own health care than is their government. According to a survey by the Consumers' Association, 40 percent of Britons surveyed would consider going to a private facility to avoid waiting, even though 84 percent of those surveyed said they did not have private medical insurance. The affluent were more willing to use private facilities, but one-third of the less well-off said they would also consider it.[9]

Astonishingly, Britain's NHS has become the largest private care provider. While large numbers of British patients waited for care, 10,000 private pay patients—about half of whom are foreign—received preferential treatment in Britain's top NHS hospitals in 2001.[10] Advertisements for one hospital boast that patients come from all over the world and the rooms are well furnished, with televisions that even have Arabic language channels.[11] An investigation by *The Observer* found that the NHS earns approximately $500 million per year in fees from treating private patients and one of the leading cancer hospitals—the Royal Marsden in London—earns one-quarter of its revenue from treating cash-paying patients.[12] Ironically, while NHS provides preferential services to patients who can pay cash, other British patients are traveling to places such as South Africa where many procedures cost less than they do at private clinics and hospitals in Britain.[13]

CANADIAN MEDICARE

Since Canada does not allow private health insurance for services covered by its Medicare system, Canadians who see the country's few private physicians or get treatment at a private hospital must pay most of the cost out of pocket. For example, Canadians sometimes choose to undergo cataract surgery on an outpatient basis in private clinics. Although the government will pay the surgeon's fee, private patients often pay $1,000 to $1,200 in "facilities fees" to obtain faster treatment than they can get at a government facility.[14]

Also, attempts to find legal loopholes in the prohibition against private pay are becoming routine. We noted above Ontario's recent ban on American professional athletes paying for care at Toronto hospitals. In British Columbia, private orthopedic clinics originally set up to treat patients in cases covered by workers compensation and auto insurance (technically outside of the Medicare system) began seeing almost anyone with a checkbook. They interpreted the prohibition against patients paying for their own care literally, and accepted payment from the patients' brothers, sisters, uncles, and so forth, instead. A new law put these clinics out of business, however.[15]

There is also a budding private market in sophisticated scanning services. Private clinics that apparently skirt the law on the theory that such services are not "necessary" medical care, are booming and now constitute 10 percent of the MRI market. St. Paul's Hospital in Vancouver offers after-hours full-body scans for less than C$1,000. A Montreal clinic offers a private CT scan for C$250. Patients wait one or two weeks for these procedures, compared to six-month waits in the public sector. A private company in Vancouver that offers PET scans for C$2,500 is attracting patients from as far away as Newfoundland.[16]

Canadians paying for private care are not all wealthy. A study by the Manitoba Center for Health Policy and Evaluation found that 40 percent of the private-pay cataract surgery patients in Winnipeg were from neighborhoods with average incomes in the lowest two-fifths of the income distribution.[17]

To reduce waiting lists for cancer treatment, seven of the ten Canadian provinces are sending some of their breast and prostate cancer patients to the United States for radiation therapy.[18] Canadians spend an estimated $1 billion on care in the United States each year.[19] Sometimes the patient's home province pays the bill. In other cases, patients spend their own money.

NOTES

1. James A. Monroe, "Citizens or Shoppers? Solidarity Under Siege," *Journal of Health Politics, Policy and Law* 25, no. 5 (October 2000): 959–68.

2. Out of a population of 53 million, 6.7 million are covered by private health insurance and another one million have cash-benefit critical illness policies. See Oliver Wright, "Private Health Cover Slumps as Cost Spirals," *The Times*, September 17, 2003. Also see Caroline Richmond, "NHS Waiting Lists Have Been a Boon for Private Medicine in the UK," *Canadian Medical Association Journal* 154, no. 3 (February 1, 1996): 378–81; and Timothy Besley, John Hall and Ian Preston, "The Demand for Private Health Insurance: Do Waiting Lists Matter?" *Journal of Public Economics* 72, no. 2 (May 1, 1999): 155–81.

3. "The Evolution of Public and Private Health Care Spending in Canada, 1960–1997," Table C.2.4, Canadian Institute for Health Information, 1999. The proportion of private medical spending in Canada is currently 30 percent. See Cynthia Ramsay, "Beyond the Public-Private Debate: An Examination of Quality, Access and Cost in the Health-Care Systems of Eight Countries," Marigond Foundation, July 2001.

4. "Health: Private Health Insurance," *Year Book Australia 2003*, Australian Bureau of Statistics, January 24, 2003, table 9.29.

5. Daniel Riordan, "Health Insurance Faces a Bitter Pill," *New Zealand Herald*, January 24, 2002.

6. See Nicholas Mays and Justin Keen, "The NHS's 50th Anniversary: Will the Fudge on Equity Sustain the NHS into the Next Millennium?" *British Medical Journal* 317, no. 7150 (July 4, 1998): 66–69.

7. "NHS Patients Opt for Private Surgery," *BBC News,* January 15, 2002. The survey was conducted by Medix UK plc, an Internet service for doctors.

8. Richmond, "NHS Waiting Lists."

9. "Forty Percent Would Go Private Unless Access to NHS Improved," Consumers' Association, May 30, 2001, available at www.which.net/whatsnew/pr/may01/general/nhs.html.

10. Anthony Browne, "Scandal of NHS Beds Auction," *The Observer,* January 6, 2002.

11. Browne, "Scandal of NHS Beds Auction."

12. Anthony Browne, "Cash-Strapped NHS Hospitals Chase Private Patient 'Bonanza'," *The Observer*, December 16, 2001

13. Anthony Browne, "NHS Cases Pay for Quick Ops in South Africa," *The Observer*, March 17, 2002.

14. Carolyn DeCoster et al., "Surgical Waiting Times in Manitoba," Manitoba Centre for Health Policy and Evaluation, June 1998; and Pippa Wysong, "The Wait-

ing Game," *Medical Post* 34, no. 28 (August 25, 1998). Although Canadian Medicare covers all medically necessary services, those services considered elective in nature are often performed in private facilities. Day surgery centers perform some of the private services. For a discussion of parallel public/private systems in Canada, see Charlotte Gray, "Visions of Our Health Care Future: Is a Parallel Private System the Answer?" *Canadian Medical Association Journal* 154, no. 7 (April 1, 1996): 1084–87.

15. For a discussion of attempts to stop private clinics, see John R. Graham and Nadeem Esmail, "The BC Government is Eroding Patient's and Physicians' Rights," Fraser Institute, December 10, 2003.

16. Tom Arnold, "Canada's Medical System Lacks Many Bells and Whistles," *National Post,* November 17, 2001.

17. C. A. DeCoster and M. D. Brownell, "Private Health Care in Canada: Savior or Siren?" *Public Health Reports* 112, no. 4 (August 1997): 298–305.

18. Cardwell, "Quebec Cancer Patients to Head South"; Walker, "Alberta Centre May Soon Fly Its CA Patients South"; and Haley et al., "Guarding the Border."

19. Steven J. Katz et al., "Phantoms in the Snow: Canadians' Use of Health Care Services in the United States," *Health Affairs* 21, no. 3 (May/June 2002): 19–31. Also see Victor Dirnfeld, "The Benefits of Privatization," *Canadian Medical Association Journal* 155, no. 4 (August 15, 1996): 407–10.

Chapter Four

Outcomes

MYTH NO. 4: ALTHOUGH THE UNITED STATES SPENDS MORE PER CAPITA ON HEALTH CARE THAN COUNTRIES WITH SINGLE-PAYER NATIONAL HEALTH INSURANCE, AMERICANS DO NOT GET BETTER HEALTH CARE

This myth is often supported by reference to two facts: (1) that life expectancy is not much different among the developed countries and (2) that the U.S. infant mortality rate is one of the highest among developed countries. If the United States spends more than other countries, why don't we rate higher than the others by these indices of health outcomes? The answer is that neither statistic is a good indicator of the quality of a country's health care system. Other indicators are much more telling.

Another problem is that these comparisons involve a selective use of statistics. Although most of our readers will be familiar with America's poor ranking on infant mortality and mediocre ranking on life expectancy (because these statistics are repeated so often by the critics), we suspect that few will be familiar with figures 4.1 and 4.2. Yet, as these figures show

- The percent of American seniors reporting they are in good health (72.6 percent) is the highest of any country in the Organization for Economic Cooperation and Development (OECD); among the also-rans, the range is from 70.8 percent in Australia to less than half (47.4 percent) in Germany.
- Among those age forty-five to sixty-four who report they are in good health, Americans top out at 85.4 percent; the others range from 84.9 percent in Canada to 58.2 percent in Germany.

FIGURE 4-1

Percent of Americans Age 65+
Reporting Health as "Good"

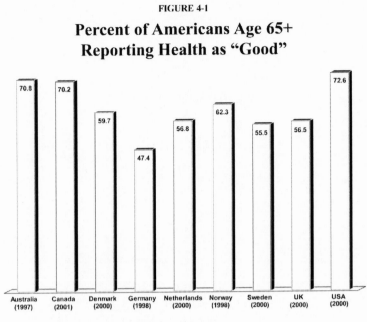

Note: Most recent data available for each country.

Source: *OECD Health Data 2002.*

FIGURE 4-2

Percent of Americans Ages 45-64
Reporting Health as "Good"

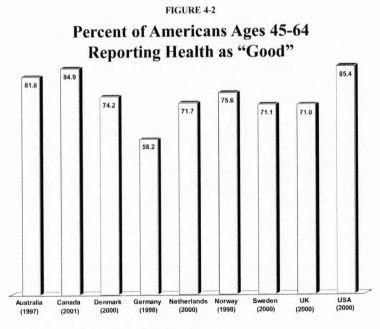

Note: Most recent data available for each country.

Source: *OECD Health Data 2002.*

Like infant mortality and life expectancy statistics, self-reported evaluations of health status may be of interest for some purposes. But these numbers are also not very good indicators of the quality of health care systems.

LIFE EXPECTANCY AND HEALTH CARE

Average life expectancy tells us almost nothing about the efficacy of health care systems because, throughout the developed world, there is very little correlation between health care spending and life expectancy. While a good health care system may, by intervention, extend the life of a small percentage of a population, it has very little to do with the average life span of the whole population. Instead, the number of years a person will live is primarily a result of genetic and social factors, including lifestyle, environment and education.[1] The American population is a mixture of ethnic groups with strikingly different expected life spans. Figures 4.3 and 4.4 show the following:

- In 1999, male life expectancy at birth ranged from 80.9 years for an Asian American, 77.2 for a Hispanic, 74.7 years for a white non-Hispanic, and 72.9 years for an American Indian down to 68.4 years for an African American.[2]
- That same year, female life expectancy ranged from 86.5 years for an Asian, 83.7 for an Hispanic, 82 years for an American Indian, and 80.1 years for a white non-Hispanic down to 75.1 years for a black.[3]

The 74.1-year life expectancy rate for the United States as a whole is a composite of these different rates. The differences between the expected life spans of groups in the United States, however, cannot be explained by differences in access to health care. Take the case of Japanese Americans. At 78.6 years, Japan has the longest life expectancy of any industrialized country, about three years longer than the United States. If the health care system were the cause of shorter life spans in the United States, one would not expect Japanese Americans to live as long as their counterparts in Japan. But they do.[4]

America is a nation of immigrants, and ethnic differences in longevity tend to persist. Thus, white Americans have life expectancy rates similar to the rates for Western Europe.[5]

INFANT MORTALITY AND HEALTH CARE

The infant mortality rate in the United States is higher than the average among developed countries at 7.2 deaths per 1,000 live births in 1998, compared to a

FIGURE 4-3

United States Life Expectancy
(Men)

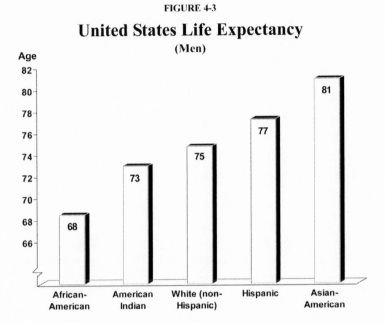

Source: National Projections Program, Population Division, U.S. Census Bureau, January 13, 2000.

FIGURE 4-4

United States Life Expectancy
(Women)

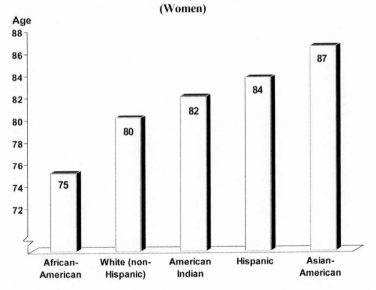

Source: *OECD Health Data 2001.*

FIGURE 4-5

Prostate Cancer Incidence and Mortality per 100,000 Males per Year

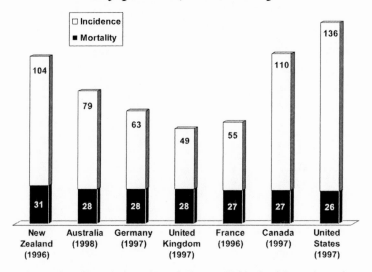

Source: Gerard F. Anderson and Peter S. Hussey, "Multinational Comparisons of Health Systems Data," Commonwealth Fund, October 2000.

Britain's third-largest city, are eight times as likely to die before reaching age four as children born in rural Gloucestershire.[25]

- Across Britain, the rate among the second lowest-income quintile ("manual classes") was 6.2 in 1999, compared to 4.3 among the highest-income quintile ("professional classes").[26]
- In the past three years alone, the rate for the lowest-income group ("unskilled manual class") has increased to double the rate of the highest-income group, a widening of nearly 10 percent.[27]

No one has seriously claimed that these differences between income groups and regions are the result of the Canadian or British health care systems. Yet, many still attempt to correlate the infant mortality rate in the United States with our health care system.

WHERE HEALTH CARE MAKES A DIFFERENCE

Although a population's general mortality is affected by many factors over which doctors and hospitals have little control, for those diseases and injuries

FIGURE 4-6

Breast Cancer Incidence and
Mortality per 100,000 Females per Year

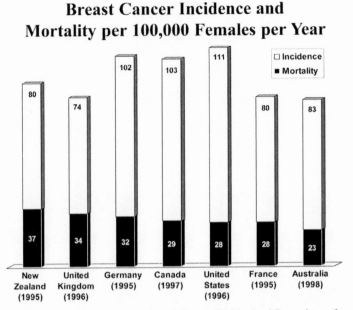

Source: Gerard F. Anderson and Peter S. Hussey, "Multinational Comparisons of
Health Systems Data, 2000," Commonwealth Fund, October 2000.

modern medicine can effectively treat, the country in which a patient lives makes a big difference. For premature babies, for children born with spina bifida or for people who have cancer, heart disease, chronic renal failure or almost any other serious illness, the chances of survival are best in the United States, where modern medical technology is most available and accessible.

Take prostate cancer, for example. In the United States, the male mortality rate for prostate cancer is slightly lower than in most other OECD countries, even though the incidence is apparently much greater (see figure 4.5). Similarly, although the incidence of breast cancer is relatively high in the United States (arguably because of lifestyle and diet), the proportion of women who die from breast cancer is among the lowest of any industrial country (see figure 4.6).

NOTES

1. "How Not To Judge Our Health Care System," National Center for Policy Analysis, Brief Analysis No. 141, November 15, 1994.

2. National Projections Program, Population Division, U.S. Census Bureau, January 13, 2000. By contrast, the 1998 figures for men in other countries are 74.8 for

Britain, 75.2 for New Zealand, 76.1 for Canada, and 76.9 for Sweden. For more information, see *OECD Health Data 2001*.

3. The 1998 figures for women in other countries are 79.7 for Britain, 80.4 for New Zealand, 81.5 for Canada, and 81.9 for Sweden. For more information, see *OECD Health Data 2001*.

4. "How Not To Judge Our Health Care System."

5. For a discussion on how life expectancy of Americans compares to that of Europeans, see Nicholas Eberstadt, *The Tyranny of Numbers: Mismeasurement & Misrule* (Washington, D.C.: American Enterprise Institute Press, 1995).

6. "Kids Count: 2001 Data Book Online," Annie E. Casey Foundation, May 17, 2002. Available at www.aecf.org; "Health, United States, 2000," National Center for Health Statistics, 2000; and *OECD Health Data 2002*.

7. The overall infant mortality rate has been falling in recent years. For example, according to OECD health data from 1998, the United States infant mortality rate fell to 7.2 per 1,000 births from 9.2 eight years earlier. The rate for the United Kingdom was 5.7 versus 7.9 eight years earlier. During the same time period, the rate in Canada dropped to 5.3 from 6.8; Australia fell to 5.0 from 8.2; and New Zealand fell to 6.8 from 8.4. See *OECD Health Data 2001*.

8. "Infant Mortality Statistics from the 1997 Period: Linked Birth/Infant Death Data Set," *National Vital Statistics Reports* 47, no. 23 (July 30, 1999).

9. *Racial and Ethnic Disparities in Infant Mortality Rates: 60 Largest U.S. Cities, 1995–1998*, Centers for Disease Control and Prevention, April 19, 2002; and *Infant Mortality: State Rankings*, National Center for Health Statistics, 2000, table 125.

10. *Racial and Ethnic Disparities in Infant Mortality Rates: 60 Largest U.S. Cities*. Also see "U.S. Childhood Mortality, 1950 through 1993: Trends and Socioeconomic Differentials," *American Journal of Public Health* 86, no. 4 (April 1996): 505–12; George A. Kaplan, "Inequality in Income and Mortality in the United States: Analysis of Mortality and Potential Pathways," *British Medical Journal* 312 (April 20, 1996): 999–1003; and Bruce P. Kennedy, "Income Distribution and Mortality: Cross-Sectional Ecological Study of the Robin Hood Index in the United States," *British Medical Journal* 312 (April 20, 1996): 1004–7.

11. Eberstadt, *The Tyranny of Numbers*. Also see "Infant Mortality, Low Birthweight and Racial Disparity in Perinatal Outcomes," National Healthy Start Association, 2001; "Healthier Mothers and Babies 1900–1999," *Journal of the American Medical Association* 282, no. 19 (November 17, 1999), 1807–1810; and "Closing the Gap: Addressing the Disparity of Infant Mortality among African-American and White Infants," Maryland Commission on Infant Mortality Prevention, 1998.

12. Eberstadt, *The Tyranny of Numbers*.

13. Eberstadt, *The Tyranny of Numbers*.

14. Eberstadt, *The Tyranny of Numbers*. On twin studies, see Olga Basso et al., "Change in Social Status and Risk of Low Birth Weight in Denmark: Population-Based Cohort Study," *British Medical Journal*, Volume 315, Issue 7121 (December 6, 1997): 1498–1502.

15. "Infant Mortality Rates and International Rankings," Centers for Disease Control and Prevention, 2001; and Eberstadt, *The Tyranny of Numbers*.

16. *OECD Health Data 2001*.

17. Eberstadt, *The Tyranny of Numbers*.

18. Eberstadt, *The Tyranny of Numbers*. The comparable rate of low birth weights for African Americans is 12.2.

19. *The Health of Canada's Children: A CICH Profile*, 2nd ed., Canadian Institute of Child Health, 1995.

20. Sheffield Health Authority reports 7.1 percent for England and Wales; North West Lancashire Health Authority reports 6.9 percent. By 2000 the latter figure had risen to 7.6 percent. See *Births, Perinatal and Infant Mortality Statistics 2000*, Health Regional Office and Health Authority of Usual Residence, UK Office of National Statistics, 2000.

21. *Medicinsk fødselstatistik* 199: *Sundhedsstatistikken* (Copenhagen: Sundhedsstyrelsen, 1995), cited in Olga Basso et al., "Change in Social Status."

22. *Births and Deaths, 1995*, Statistics Canada, Catalogue 84-210-XPB.

23. *Births and Deaths, 1995*, Statistics Canada, Catalogue 84-210-XPB. Also see R. Wilkins, "Mortality by Neighborhood Income in Urban Canada, 1986–1991," presentation to the Canadian Society for Epidemiology and Biostatistics, St. John's, Newfoundland, August 1995.

24. *Births and Deaths, 1995*, Statistics Canada, Catalogue 84-210-XPB.

25. Daniel Dorling, "Death in Britain: How Local Mortality Rates Have Changed," Policy Brief Report, Joseph Roundtree Foundation, 1997.

26. "Health Inequalities—National Targets on Infant Mortality and Life Expectancy," *Health Statistics Quarterly*, no. 12, November 2001.

27. "Health Inequalities—National Targets."

Chapter Five

Technology

MYTH NO. 5: COUNTRIES WITH
SINGLE-PAYER NATIONAL HEALTH CARE
SYSTEMS HAVE ACCESS TO THE LATEST TECHNOLOGY

One could argue that the need for technology varies from country to country. For example, the incidence of AIDS, breast cancer and prostate cancer is higher in the United States than in many other developed countries[1] (see figure 5.1). However, every country needs certain critical, lifesaving technologies to diagnose and treat disease. A nation's ability and willingness to sufficiently invest in modern medical technology is one determinant of the effectiveness of its health care system. By this measure, the United States fares better than its single-payer counterparts.[2]

THE POLITICS OF MEDICAL TECHNOLOGY

Overall, the best way to think about government policies toward technology is in terms of the politics of medicine. As the role of government expands, health care tends to evolve from a protechnology phase to an antitechnology phase. In the first stage, government tends to spend on items perceived as underprovided by the market or by conventional health insurance. Thus, practically every less-developed country has used government funds to build at least one modern hospital, usually in the largest city, and to stock it with at least one example of each new technology, while all but the wealthiest citizens lack basic medical care and public sanitation.

FIGURE 5-1

Incidence of Disease

(Per 100,000 people per year)

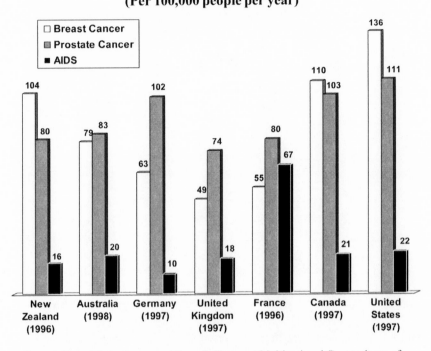

Source: Gerard F. Anderson and Peter S. Hussey, "Multinational Comparisons of
Health Systems Data," Commonwealth Fund, October 2000.

As government's role in medicine expands, more and more interest groups
must be accommodated. In this stage, government policy tends to become antitechnology because the few people who are acutely or chronically ill and need
expensive technology are heavily outnumbered by the healthier many who desire amenities. (The nature of these amenities will be discussed in detail in chapter 11.) Along the way, these general trends may be violated with respect to any
particular technology because of the varied, even random, ways in which special
interest pressures are exerted. (We will return to the politics of medicine below.)

USE OF MODERN MEDICAL PROCEDURES

As a result of these political pressures, patients in countries with single-payer
health systems usually have less access to critical medical procedures. Figure

FIGURE 5-2

Use of High-Tech Medical Procedures

(Procedures per 100,000 people per year)

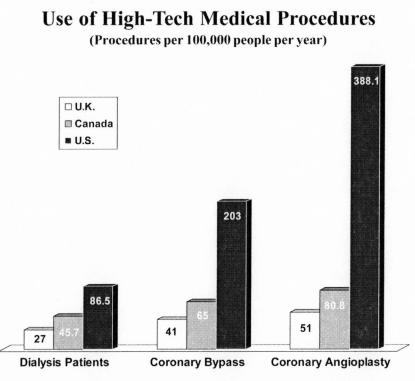

Source: Gerard F. Anderson, Uwe E. Reinhardt, Peter S. Hussey and Varduhi
Petrosyan, "It's the Prices, Stupid: Why the United States Is So
Different from Other Countries," *Health Affairs*, Vol. 22, No. 3, May/
June 2003: 89–105

5.2 compares the rate of use for high-tech medical procedures in Britain,
Canada and the United States:

• The use of coronary bypass surgery in the United States is slightly more
than three times higher per capita than in Canada and almost five times
higher than in Britain.
• The rate of coronary angioplasty in the United States is almost five times
higher than in Canada and almost eight times higher than Britain's.
• The rate of renal dialysis in the United States is almost double that of
Canada and more than three times that of Britain.

ACCESS TO MEDICAL TECHNOLOGY IN BRITAIN

Although Britain has pioneered the development of important medical technology, the British often have less access to that technology than patients in other countries. For example, Britain was the codeveloper with the United States of kidney dialysis in the 1970s, yet Britain consistently has had one of the lowest dialysis rates in Europe. According to British renal specialists, today the country has only enough kidney dialysis capability to meet 82 percent of the need,[3] which implies that one in eight Britons who need kidney treatment do not receive it. However, British doctors may be underestimating the need, perhaps because they are conditioned by the culture of rationing. As we saw in figure 5.2, the number of people accepted for renal therapy per capita in the United States is more than three times that of Britain. Computed tomography (CT) scanners, which are useful in the diagnosis and treatment of cancer,[4] were also invented in Britain. For years Britain manufactured and exported about half the CT scanners used in the world. Yet, through the years the British government purchased very few scanners for the NHS, and even discouraged private gifts of the devices to the NHS.[5] Today Britain has only half the number of CT scanners per million population (6.5) as the United States (13.6).[6]

While critics of the U.S. health care system claim that we have too much technology, all the evidence suggests that our counterparts have too little as a result of the conscious decisions of government officials. As figure 5.3 shows, Britain's NHS has also skimped on the newer magnetic resonance imaging (MRI) scanners that can detect disease throughout the body, including aneurysms or tears in the aorta, strokes and tumors. Britain (at 3.9 MRI scanners per million population) has less than half as many as the United States (8.1 per million). There is strong evidence of a general underuse of other valuable therapies as well.[7] For instance,

- An Institute of Economic Affairs study argues that one effect of underinvestment in technology is that Britain has the lowest survival rates for victims of lung cancer and heart disease among European countries.[8]
- ACE inhibitors, used in coronary heart failure, are prescribed to only 20 percent to 30 percent of patients with heart failure.[9]
- Echocardiography, a diagnostic test that uses ultrasound waves to make images of the heart, is not available to all patients, although it is low-cost and highly effective; in some regions only about one-third of heart failure patients receive it.[10]

Not only is the heart disease survival rate poor in Britain, the country is doing little to improve it; a British Cardiac Society survey found risk factors management and preventive treatment to be well short of what they should be.[11]

FIGURE 5-3

Access to Modern Medical Technology in the U.S., Britain and Canada (2000)

(Units per million people)

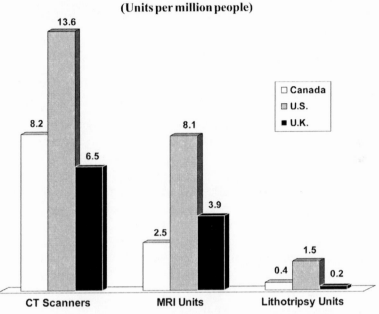

Sources: Gerard F. Anderson, Uwe E. Reinhardt, Peter S. Hussey and Varduhi Petrosyan, "It's the Prices, Stupid: Why the United States is So Different from Other Countries," *Health Affairs*, Vol. 22, No. 3, May/June 2003, Exhibit 5, p. 97; and Stephen Pollard, "European Health Care Consensus Group Paper," Centre for the New Europe, January 4, 2001.

ACCESS TO MODERN MEDICAL TECHNOLOGY IN CANADA

In terms of availability of advanced medical technology, Canada now ranks at the bottom of the twenty-nine OECD countries, despite the fact that Canadian spending on health care (as a percentage of GDP) is fifth in the world.[12] Figure 5.3 compares the availability of modern medical technology in the United States, Britain and Canada:

- On a per capita basis, the United States has more than three times as many MRI units as Canada.[13]
- Per person, the United States has nearly four times as many lithotripsy units, which avoid expensive and invasive surgery by using sound waves to destroy kidney stones and gallstones.[14]

- The United States has almost twice as many CT scanners per capita as Canada.[15]
- As of November 2001, Canada had only 3 public-sector PET scanners—and one of those only operated one evening a week—compared to 250 in the United States.[16]

In addition, much of the medical technology that is available in Canada is archaic and ineffective. In Canadian hospitals, for example, 63 percent of all general X-ray equipment is severely outdated and half of all diagnostic imaging units require replacement.[17]

At the regional level, the difference in the level of access Americans and Canadians have to such technologies is even more striking. Figure 5.4 shows the percentage of hospitals in British Columbia, Washington and Oregon that are equipped to provide specialized services. As the figure shows, in 1999[18]

- Angioplasty, a procedure to dilate obstructed coronary arteries, was available at only one regional hospital in British Columbia, compared to 80 percent of the facilities in Washington and Oregon.
- Cardiac catheterization, which assesses the extent of blockage in coronary arteries, was available at only 20 percent of the hospitals in British Columbia, but is widely available south of the border.

There also is a wide difference in the availability of other technologies.[19]

- In the state of Washington, virtually 100 percent of community and regional hospitals have access to MRI units, compared to 20 percent in neighboring British Columbia.
- In the state of Oregon, 90 percent of community and regional hospitals have access to lithotripsy units, while there are none whatsoever in British Columbia.

Theoretically, Canadians are not allowed to purchase MRI scans, despite long waits in the public sector. Yet, as we have seen, loopholes in the law are being tested as private scanning clinics pop up around the country, similar to what has happened in the United States. Americans not only pay out of pocket for MRI scans, they do not even need a doctor's order or any indication of a medical problem. Indeed, for $500 or so, U.S. citizens can purchase full body scans at shopping malls much as they engage in other impulse buying. Although the medical community tends to be scornful, there is the odd chance that a scan may save a person's life, much as the purchase of a flashlight might save a person's life.

FIGURE 5-4

Availability of Medical Technology in British Columbia, Washington & Oregon Hospitals

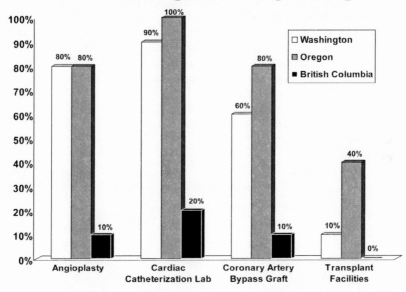

Source: David Harriman, William McArthur and Martin Zelder, "The Availability of Medical Technology in Canada: An International Comparative Study," Fraser Institute, 1999.

NOTES

1. Anderson and Hussey, "Multinational Comparisons of Health Systems Data," Commonwealth Fund.

2. Uwe Reinhardt, Peter S. Hussey and Gerard F. Anderson, "Cross-National Comparisons of Health Systems Using OECD Data, 1999," *Health Affairs* 21, no. 3 (May/June 2002): 169–81, Exhibit 5.

3. David Green and Laura Casper, *Delay, Denial and Dilution: The Impact of NHS Rationing on Heart Disease and Cancer* (London: Institute of Economic Affairs, 2000).

4. "Health and Medical Information," *MedicineNet.com.* Accessed December 2003.

5. John C. Goodman, *National Health Care in Great Britain: Lessons for the U.S.A.* (Dallas: Fisher Institute, 1980), 96–104.

6. Gerard F. Anderson, Uwe E. Reinhardt, Peter S. Hussey, and Varduhi Petrosyan, "It's the Prices, Stupid: Why the United States Is So Different from Other Countries," *Health Affairs* 22, no. 3 (May/June 2003): 89–105.

7. For a framework of NHS coronary care goals, see "National Service Framework for Coronary Heart Disease," UK Department of Health, London, 2000.

8. Green and Casper, *Delay, Denial and Dilution.*

9. Green and Casper, *Delay, Denial and Dilution.* ACE inhibitors lower blood pressure by blocking Angiotensin Converting Enzyme, which allows blood vessels to relax and expand. Also see Martin Eccles, Nick Freemantle and James Mason, "North of England Evidence-Based Development Project: Guideline for Angiotensin Converting Enzyme Inhibitors in Primary Care Management of Adults with Symptomatic Heart Failure," *British Medical Journal* 316 (May 2, 1998): 1369–75.

10. Green and Casper, *Delay, Denial and Dilution.*

11. Green and Casper, *Delay, Denial and Dilution.*

12. David Harriman, William McArthur and Martin Zelder, "The Availability of Medical Technology in Canada: An International Comparative Study," Fraser Institute, Public Policy Sources No. 28, August 6, 1999.

13. Anderson et al., "It's the Prices, Stupid."

14. Pollard, "European Health Care Consensus Group Paper." For a comparison of OECD countries, also see Harriman, McArthur and Zelder, "The Availability of Medical Technology in Canada."

15. Anderson et al., "It's the Prices, Stupid."

16. Tom Arnold, "Canada's Medical System Lacks Many Bells and Whistles," *National Post*, November 17, 2001.

17. Canadian Association of Radiologists. Reported in Tom Arnold, "X-ray Labs Dangerously Outdated," *National Post*, October 12, 2000.

18. Harriman, McArthur and Zelder, "The Availability of Medical Technology in Canada."

19. Harriman, McArthur and Zelder, "The Availability of Medical Technology in Canada."

Chapter Six

Quality

MYTH NO. 6: COUNTRIES WITH SINGLE-PAYER NATIONAL HEALTH CARE SYSTEMS HAVE A HIGHER QUALITY OF HEALTH CARE THAN THE UNITED STATES

Proponents of a single-payer system for the United States maintain it would "provide access to high-quality care for everyone at an affordable price."[1] To support this idea, some point to a report comparing health systems in countries worldwide, published by the World Health Organization (WHO). However, the WHO report does not support the claim that single-payer health insurance leads to high-quality care.

INTERNATIONAL COMPARISON: THE WHO REPORT

In 2000 the WHO issued a report comparing health care systems in 191 countries.[2] In the overall WHO ranking, the French health care system ranked first. The U.S. system ranked thirty-seventh, just above Slovenia (38) and below Costa Rica (36).

Rest assured. Americans are not boarding planes bound for Costa Rica—or even for France—in search of better health care. Still, officials in other countries have used the report to argue that their health systems are not as bad as their citizens might suspect. And some politicians in the United States have used the report to support their claim that American health care needs even more government intervention and control.

So what's wrong with the WHO report? What's wrong is that it mainly reflects perceptions of fairness and equity rather than success at saving lives and curing diseases.

The WHO report ranks nations with respect to "overall health system performance" based on five factors, using data from the OECD and WHO surveys of the opinions of experts and officials in those countries. The five factors (and their weighting in the overall scores) were the level of health (25 percent); the equal distribution of health indicators by income and/or ethnic group (25 percent); the responsiveness of the system to patient needs—including the level of responsiveness (12.5 percent) and the distribution of responsiveness by income and/or ethnic group (12.5 percent); and the fairness of the country's financing (25 percent), which measures how much more, as a portion of income, higher-income groups pay for their health care than lower-income groups.

These measures produced some odd, almost random rankings. For example:

- Japan ranked first on the attainment of health, measured in Disability Adjusted Life Expectancy (DALE), but Chile ranked first in the equal distribution of DALE among subgroups.
- The United States ranked first in the responsiveness of its system, but the United Arab Emirates (UAE) ranked first in the distribution of responsiveness.
- Colombia ranked first in the fairness of its health system financing.

As we discussed previously, the overall health of a country's population is strongly influenced by its demographic makeup. Thus, it makes sense that Japan, with low infant mortality and greater life spans, ranks first in terms of overall healthiness. But beyond some basic public health measures, there is not much correlation internationally between health care inputs and the overall health of a population.

Of the five measures used to calculate the overall WHO ranking, only health system responsiveness takes patients into account. And even this ranking was not based on objective data. It was based instead on patient surveys and surveys of officials and experts in each country with regard to "(a) respect for persons (including dignity, confidentiality and autonomy of individuals and families to decide about their own health); and (b) client orientation (including prompt attention, access to social support networks during care, quality of basic amenities and choice of provider)."

On that measure, the United States ranked first. But so what? Respect and amenities are nice. But what about life saving treatment? In most people's minds that matters much more.

FIGURE 6-1

How Sicker Patients
Evaluate Their Health Care

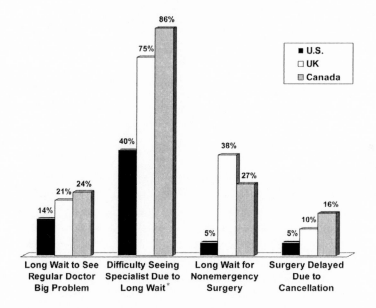

* Note: Sample was of those who reported difficulty seeing specialist.

Sources: Robert J. Blendon, et al., "Inequities in Health Care: A Five-Country Survey,"
    Health Affairs, Vol. 21, No. 3, May/June 2002: 182-191; Robert J. Blendon et al.,
    "Common Concerns Amid Diverse Systems: Health Care Experiences in Five
    Countries," *Health Affairs*, Vol. 22, No. 3, May/June 2003: 106-121.

INTERNATIONAL COMPARISON:
THE COMMONWEALTH FUND SURVEYS

While the WHO rankings are mainly based on what people think is fair, a series of Commonwealth Fund surveys asked patients about their actual health care. In particular, the surveys asked patients and "sicker" adults, most of whom described their health as "fair" or "poor," in several countries to rate the performance of their nation's health care system.[3] Figure 6.1 shows the following:

- Only 14 percent in the United States cited long waits to see their regular doctor as a "big problem," compared to 21 percent in the United Kingdom and 24 percent in Canada.[4]

- Among those experiencing difficulties seeing a specialist, 40 percent in the United States reported difficulty due to a long waiting list, compared to 75 percent in the United Kingdom and 86 percent in Canada.[5]
- Only 5 percent in the United States reported long waits for nonemergency surgery, compared to 27 percent in Canada and 38 percent in the UK.[6]
- Only 5 percent in the United States reported a surgery delayed due to a cancellation, compared to 10 percent in the United Kingdom and 16 percent in Canada.[7]

QUALITY PROBLEMS IN CANADA

Canada's federal health care payments to the provinces were slashed after the 1995–1996 budget year. Many hospitals were closed or consolidated.[8] Waiting periods for patients facing life-threatening conditions grew as a result and the effects have been severe. Whereas the Canadian Society of Surgical Oncology recommends that cancer treatment, including surgery, begin within two weeks after preoperative tests, one study found that the median wait was much longer. Depending on the type of cancer, the median waiting time for surgery varied from almost a month (29.0 days) for colorectal cancer to more than two months (64.0 days) for urologic cancers.[9]

The frustration felt by physicians who witnessed first hand the deteriorating standards of care in Canada's hospitals is apparent in a survey conducted by the Canadian Medical Association. Of physicians surveyed, only 27 percent rated their access to advanced diagnostic services as excellent, very good or good. Fewer than two-thirds rated their access to acute care when urgently needed as excellent, very good or good.[10]

The Canadian press is replete with the names of the victims of rationing or inadequate care. Among the cases reported,

- It took four hours for a Toronto critical care specialty referral service to find an available hospital bed for Jeyaraanie Kaneshakumar, a pregnant woman who collapsed in her suburban Scarborough home from a brain hemorrhage. She died.[11]
- A Toronto man who fell ill while vacationing in Rhode Island was forced to stay in an American hospital for six weeks because no bed could be found for him in Ontario. A free bed was located only after the media exposed the man's plight.[12]
- Dan Smith of Brampton, Ontario, was denied a double lung transplant—his only hope for survival—when his surgery was cancelled due to a bed shortage in intensive care units (ICUs). A pair of donated lungs was wasted, although thirty other Ontarians were also waiting for lung transplants.[13]

- Kyle Martyn, a five-year old boy taken to the emergency room with toxic shock waited three hours to see a doctor. The ER was backlogged because three-fourths of its beds were occupied with patients awaiting transfer to acute care beds. The acute care beds were full of "bed blockers" who had nowhere to go due to the shortage of long-term care beds. Kyle died from complications.[14]

QUALITY PROBLEMS IN BRITAIN

In an extensive study of Britain's NHS in the mid-1980s, Brookings Institution economists estimated the number of British patients denied treatment each year, based on U.S. levels of treatment. Most of the patients suffered from life-threatening diseases and the denial of treatment meant certain death. According to the study,[15]

- About 9,000 British kidney patients failed to receive renal dialysis or a kidney transplant—and presumably died as a result.
- As many as 15,000 cancer patients and 17,000 heart patients failed to receive the best treatment.
- As many as 1,000 British children failed to receive lifesaving total parenteral nutrition (TPN) therapy and about 7,000 elderly patients were denied pain-relieving hip replacements.

Although the study has not been updated, casual observation suggests that the difference between US and British levels of care have widened rather than narrowed over the past twenty years. Take kidney dialysis, for example.[16] The number of dialysis patients per 100,000 Britons is only about one-third the rate in the United States, although the prevalence of kidney disease is not much different.[17] One in eight British nephrologists say that due to limited resources they have refused treatment to patients they thought were suitable for such care.[18] The comparable figure among United States nephrologists is 2 percent.

NHS officials are repeatedly embarrassed by the popular press. Britons are now more likely to be killed by an infection caught in a hospital than by a car accident, claimed a BBC broadcast based on a leaked government report.[19] Like the Canadian media, the British media teems with reports of patients harmed by inadequate care:

- Nine-year-old Tony Clowes, in a hospital to have the tip of his right index finger reattached after a bicycle chain accident, died under anesthesia from lack of oxygen when a breathing tube became blocked. The $1.50 tube, designed for one use only, had been reused for six weeks to reduce costs.[20]

- George Mitchell Sr., 73, who was undergoing treatment for bladder cancer at Scotland's biggest cancer treatment center, was sent off in a taxi to a hotel with no access to medical care before the treatment was finished because the hospital was short of beds. Hospital officials said it was a mistake.[21]
- Britain's Audit Commission said hospital pharmacies lack the computer systems needed to keep pace with modern medicine. Consequently, in England and Wales, five times more patients died in 2000 from receiving the wrong medicine than a decade earlier.[22]

COMPARING MORTALITY RATES

As we discussed previously, a country's overall mortality rate isn't much affected by its health system. The mortality rate for certain conditions is very much affected by the quality of care, however. In countries where governments control health care resources, patients do not always receive the treatment they need or they may be denied access to the most effective treatment.

Take cancer mortality rates, for example. As figure 6.2 illustrates, in New Zealand and the United Kingdom nearly half of all women diagnosed with

FIGURE 6-2

Breast Cancer Mortality Ratio
(Percent of those with the disease who die from it)

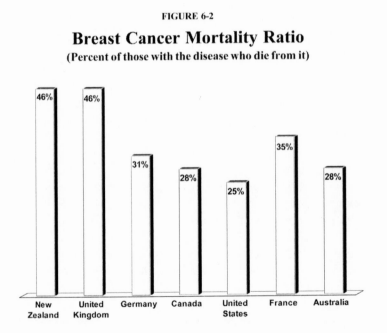

Source: Gerard F. Anderson and Peter S. Hussey, "Multinational Comparisons of Health Systems Data," Commonwealth Fund, October 2000.

breast cancer die of the disease. In Germany and France, almost one in three die. By contrast, in the United States only one in four women diagnosed with breast cancer dies.

In the United States, slightly less than one in five men diagnosed with prostate cancer dies of the disease. In the United Kingdom, 57 percent die. France and Germany fare slightly better at 49 percent and 44 percent, respectively. At 30 percent and 25 percent, respectively, death rates from prostate cancer in New Zealand and Canada are still well above those of the United States (see figure 6.3).

Overall, the annual rate of cancer deaths is 70 percent higher in the United Kingdom than in the United States—275 deaths per 100,000 and 194 deaths per 100,000, respectively.[23] Indeed, a WHO study calculated that 25,000 people die unnecessarily in Britain each year because they are denied the highest quality of cancer care.[24]

FIGURE 6-3

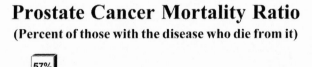

Prostate Cancer Mortality Ratio
(Percent of those with the disease who die from it)

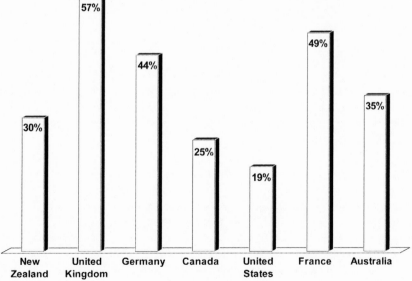

Source: Gerard F. Anderson and Peter S. Hussey, "Multinational Comparisons of Health Systems Data," Commonwealth Fund, October 2000.

QUALITY PROBLEMS IN THE UNITED STATES

There are also quality problems in the United States. Several studies have identified a rate of hospital injury—due to negligence or treatment errors—of approximately 0.92 percent of admissions. Nationally, that translates into about 300,000 patients injured each year.[25] In 1999 the Institute of Medicine reported that between 44,000 and 98,000 patients die each year of medical errors.[26] Some of these incidents are widely reported. Linda McDougal, 46, was diagnosed with an aggressive form of breast cancer and doctors performed a double radical mastectomy at a St. Paul, Minnesota, hospital. Days after the surgery, her doctor revealed that her test results had been switched with another women's, and she had no cancer.[27] A Rhode Island surgeon operated on the wrong side of a patient's head after a CT scan was placed backward on an X-ray viewing box. The surgical site had not been marked with a pen as hospital policy required.[28] However unfortunate such surgical errors are, they appear to be unusual.[29]

The United States shares some quality problems with the systems of other developed countries because of a common defect noted in the Introduction: all developed countries have suppressed normal market forces. As a result, in health care we do not observe the quality control we have come to expect in profit-making enterprises. Indeed, all over the developed world hospitals lack the quality controls observable in corner supermarkets.[30] In this respect, differences between the United States and other countries are differences of degree. We note parenthetically, however, that the United States is more aggressively pushing its hospital sector to adopt business techniques for managing quality.

In other respects, differences between the U.S. health care system and the systems of other countries are differences of kind. Although mistakes are made in U.S. hospitals, patients are not routinely denied access to lifesaving drugs and lifesaving technology, as happens elsewhere around the world.

NOTES

1. Don R. McCanne, "Would Single-Payer Health Insurance Be Good for America?" Physicians for a National Health Program, March 27, 2000.

2. *The World Health Report 2000—Health Systems: Improving Performance* (World Health Organization, 2000).

3. Sample population is "sicker" and is likely to rate health as "fair" or "poor." New Zealand had the least unhealthy sample, 38 percent of sample rating their health "fair" or "poor." The United Kingdom had the most unhealthy sample with 62 percent rating their health "fair" or "poor."

4. Robert J. Blendon, Cathy Schoen, Catherine DesRoches, Robin Osborn, and Kinga Zapert, "Common Concerns Amid Diverse Systems: Health Care Experiences in Five Countries," *Health Affairs* 22, no. 3 (May/June 2003): 106–21.

5. Blendon et al., "Common Concerns Amid Diverse Systems."

6. Robert J. Blendon, Cathy Schoen, Catherine M. DesRoches, Robin Osborn, Kimberly L. Scoles, and Kinga Zapert, "Inequities in Health Care: A Five-Country Survey," *Health Affairs* 21, no. 3 (May/June 2002): 182–91.

7. Blendon et al., "Common Concerns Amid Diverse Systems," 106–21.

8. "Ottawa Eyes Cure for Health Funding," *Toronto Star*, November 4, 1997.

9. Marko Simunovic et al., "A Snapshot of Waiting Times for Cancer Surgery Provided by Surgeons Affiliated with Regional Cancer Centres in Ontario," *Canadian Medical Association Journal* 165, no. 4 (August 21, 2001): 421–25.

10. "Physician Resource Questionnaire," Canadian Medical Association, January 1998; and Canadian Medical Association, "Canadians' Access to Quality Health Care: A System in Crisis," submitted to the House of Commons Standing Committee on Finance, August 31, 1998.

11. Kellie Hudson, "Patient's Death 'Anomaly': Despite Futile Bed Search; Agency Says System Works but Doctors Disagree," *Toronto Star*, July 3, 1998.

12. Siri Agrell, "Toronto Bed Found for Man Who Fell Ill in U.S.," *National Post*, August 8, 2003.

13. Vince Talotta, "The Sickness in Our Health System," *Toronto Star*, February 6, 1999.

14. "The Boy Who Ran Out of Time," *Toronto Star*, December 12, 1999.

15. Author's calculations based on Henry J. Aaron and William B. Schwartz, *The Painful Prescription: Rationing Hospital Care* (Washington, D.C.: Brookings Institution, 1984). Reported in John C. Goodman and Gerald L. Musgrave, "Twenty Myths about National Health Insurance," NCPA Policy Report No. 128, National Center for Policy Analysis, December 1991.

16. Although its population is about one-sixth that of the United States, the United Kingdom spends less than 6 percent as much on treatment of renal failure, or less than $1 billion per year compared to more than $17 billion in the United States. Figures reported in British pounds were converted to U.S. dollars. See Sheffield Kidney Research Foundation, Background to SKRF, available at www.skrf.org.uk/background.html. Accessed December 4, 2003.

17. Gerard F. Anderson, Uwe E. Reinhardt, Peter S. Hussey, and Varduhi Petrosyan, "It's the Prices, Stupid: Why the United States Is So Different from Other Countries," *Health Affairs* 22, no. 3 (May/June 2003): Exhibit 6. See also E. C. Mulkerrin, "Rationing Renal Replacement Therapy to Older Patients: Agreed Guidelines Are Needed," *QJ Med* 93, no. 4 (April 2000): 253–55.

18. J. K. Mackenzie et al., "Dialysis Decision Making in Canada, the United Kingdom, and the United States," *American Journal of Kidney Diseases* 31, no. 1 (1998): 12–18. Britain, at 12 percent, was only slightly worse than Canada, where 10 percent of nephrologists report refusing treatment due to limited resources.

19. "Watchdog Healthcheck," *BBC Online News,* January 15, 2001. Research by the Public Health Laboratory Service and the London School of Hygiene and Tropical

Medicine set the cost of hospital-acquired infections at £1 billion. The National Audit Office estimates that as many as 5,000 people die each year of the infections. See "Hospital Infections Cost £1 Billion a Year," *BBC News,* January 18, 2000; and "NHS Bugs Kill 5,000 a Year," *BBC News*, February 17, 2000.

20. Olga Craig, "'How Could Someone Look Down at My Little Boy and End His Life, in a Hospital, Where He Should Be Safe?'" *Sunday Telegraph* (London), August 19, 2001.

21. Aine Harrington, "Beatson Put Dying Man in a Hotel; Son Tells of Father Being Moved 'from Pillar to Post,'" *Glasgow Herald*, November 16, 2001.

22. Lorna Duckworth, "Obsolete Systems Blamed for Rise in NHS Drug Deaths," *The Independent*, December 18, 2001.

23. This may be partially due to the fact that the NHS spends much less on treatment—$1.35 per capita compared to $24.35 per capita in the United States. Nick Bosanquet, "A Successful NHS: From Aspiration to Delivery," Adam Smith Institute, 1999, 10.

24. Karol Sikora, "Cancer Survival in Britain," *British Medical Journal* (August 21, 1999): 461–62.

25. Elise C. Becher and Mark Chassin, "Improving the Quality of Health Care: Who Will Lead?" *Health Affairs* 20, no. 5 (September/October 2001): 164–79.

26. Institute of Medicine, *To Err Is Human: Building a Safer Health Care System* (Washington, D.C.: National Academy Press, 1999).

27. "Mastectomy Mistake Fuels Debate," *CBSNews.com,* January 21, 2003.

28. "Protect Yourself from Wrong Site Surgery," Employer Health Care Alliance Cooperative, available at www.alliancehealthcoop.com. Accessed December 12, 2003.

29. The sentinel event database of the Joint Commission on Accreditation of Healthcare Organizations lists a total of 232 wrong site surgeries from 1995 to October 28, 2003. "Sentinel Event Statistics: As of October 28, 2003," Joint Commission on Accreditation of Healthcare Organizations, available at www.jcaho.org. Accessed December 12, 2003.

30. About 125 of the more than 5,000 hospitals in the United States used supermarket-style bar code systems to identify drugs and vials of blood in 2003. A 2004 Federal Food and Drug Administration order was expected to require bar codes on medications sold to hospitals. See Lauren Neergaard, "New Rules Expected to Reduce Deaths from Medication Errors," *Associated Press/Dallas Morning News*, December 17, 2003.

Chapter Seven

Costs

MYTH NO. 7: COUNTRIES WITH SINGLE-PAYER NATIONAL HEALTH CARE SYSTEMS HAVE BEEN MORE SUCCESSFUL THAN THE UNITED STATES IN CONTROLLING HEALTH CARE COSTS

The United States spends more on health care than any other country in the world, both in dollars per person and as a percentage of GDP. Does this mean that our predominantly private health care system is less able to control spending than are developed countries with national health insurance? Not necessarily.

As we shall see, international comparisons of health care spending are difficult, not least because of differences in the measuring techniques used by other countries.[1] First, however, we should note that the United States is wealthier than other countries. Almost without exception, international comparisons show that wealthier countries spend a larger proportion of their GDP on health care.[2] In his classic 1977 and 1981 studies, health economist Joseph Newhouse found that 90 percent of the variation in health care spending among developed countries is based on income alone.[3] This should give pause to anyone who believes that the United States will significantly lower health care spending by adopting the system or institutions of some other country. As we noted in the introduction, as people have more income, they spend more on health care, whether their spending takes place through the market, the political system or quasipublic institutions.

Some believe that countries with national single-payer health insurance have a coercive "advantage" the United States does not—they can more easily deny access to care. Governments, for example, can and do limit health care dollars and force hospitals and doctors to ration services. However, such power is not unlimited. Politicians who abuse it risk being replaced by their competitors. In the political systems of other countries, just as in the United States, the pressure to spend more on health care is unrelenting.

THE UNITED STATES VERSUS
OTHER DEVELOPED COUNTRIES

Most international statistics on health care spending are produced by the OECD. However, OECD statistics are not always useful because different countries use different methods to report costs.[4] No effective international guidelines exist, and some countries include services that others do not.[5] For instance, the OECD definition of health care expenditures includes nursing home care. But while Germany includes nursing home care as part of total health expenditures, Britain does not.[6] Some countries count hospital beds simply by counting metal frames with mattresses, whether or not they are in use. In others, a "bed" is counted only if it is staffed and operational.[7]

Although the percentage of the population admitted as inpatients in the United States (11.8) is below the OECD average of 15.4 percent, the U.S. figures exclude procedures performed in outpatient facilities, while OECD figures most likely include these surgeries.[8] In addition, payments made in the "informal health sector" (under-the-table payments, common in many countries) are generally missed in official estimates.[9]

Figure 7.1 shows the result of an attempt to develop more accurate health care spending measurements among OECD countries. The study calculated the average annual increase in the percentage of per capita spending on health care by OECD countries for the period 1960 to 1998. As the figure shows, the countries of the OECD have been no more successful than the United States in controlling costs and many have been far less successful. During the 1990s, health care spending in all but three of fifteen OECD countries studied grew at about the same rate as in the United States—or higher. The real rate of expenditures on hospital and physician services actually decreased in the United States in the 1990s (2.5 percent and 1.0 percent, respectively), well below the OECD median for both categories.[10]

These results are surprising considering that the United States has far less rationing of care and offers greater access to medical technology. Furthermore, the United States confronts a wider range of health problems than most other OECD countries. For example, the incidence of AIDS is almost ten times more prevalent in the United States than in Canada, and obesity is a greater problem here than in other developed countries (see figure 7.2).[11] These factors, of course, put greater demands on the U.S. health care system.

FIGURE 7-1

Average Annual Real Growth in
Per Capita Health Spending
1960-1998

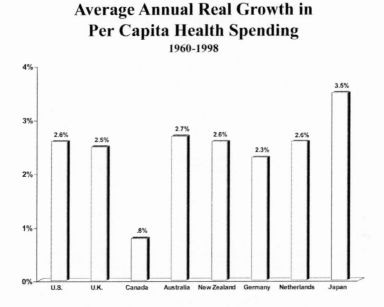

Source: Gerard F. Anderson et al., "Health Spending and Outcomes: Trends in OECD
Countries, 1960-1998," *Health Affairs*, May/June 2000.

FIGURE 7-2

Percent of the Population Age 15
and Older That Is Obese

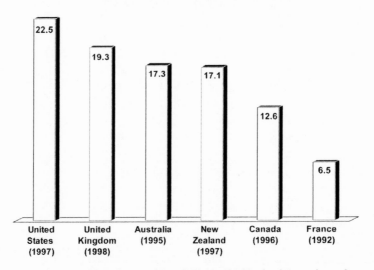

Source: Gerard F. Anderson and Peter S. Hussey, "Multinational Comparisons of
Health Systems Data," Commonwealth Fund, October 2000.

THE UNITED STATES VERSUS CANADA

During the 1990s, Canada was able to limit the real rate of growth in its health care spending to 1.7 percent per year. By contrast, the rate of spending growth in the United States health care system was equal to the OECD median of 3.0 percent per year.[12] However, as we document elsewhere in this book, Canada limited spending increases by cutting funding for services in ways that caused people to suffer.

• The Canadian federal government reduced block grants to provinces for health care as a percentage of GDP in 1986 and again in 1989; funding to the provinces was frozen at 1989–1990 levels through 1995, and further cuts were made in the second half of the 1990s.[13]
• Provincial governments, in turn, reduced funding available to hospitals (their global budgets), began limiting total expenditures for physicians' fees, severely limited the purchase of new technology, and removed some services from coverage by provincial insurance plans.[14]
• Many smaller hospitals were closed—fifty in Saskatchewan alone—and the number of hospital beds available nationwide was reduced from 6.6 per thousand population in 1987 to 4.1 in 1995.[15]

By most accounts, these reductions in the availability of medical services had more to do with budgetary shortfalls than lack of medical need. A recent report for the Canadian federal government argued that the Canadian health care system was under funded and in need of an additional C$5 billion annually.[16] Satisfaction with the Canadian health care system fell throughout the 1990s as a result. As we have seen, when medical resources are allocated based on limited global budgets, patients often go without needed care.

In 2000, the United States spent 13.0 percent of its GDP, or US $4,631 per person, on health care. By contrast, Canada spent 9.1 percent of its GDP, or US $2,535 per person.[17] Here again, the spending figures are almost certainly incomplete. In both Canada and the United States, the costs of administering government health care spending are largely hidden. In addition, there are larger, systemic differences between the two countries:[18]

• Canadian figures do not include the capital cost of building and equipment to the extent that the U.S. figures do because Canadian facilities are paid for by the government; hence, the cost of capital is subsumed within the Canadian government's debt.
• The United States spends far more on research and development (R&D) than Canada. The U.S. spending results in technological innovations that benefit Canada and the rest of the world.

- The U.S. population is slightly older, and older people inevitably consume more health care.

According to one study, correcting for these differences between the two countries cuts in half the gap in the fraction of GDP spent on health care.[19]

In addition to AIDS and obesity, the United States has other demands on its health care system that Canada does not. For example, the U.S. male homicide rate is three times that of Canada.[20] The United States also has health care costs related to war injuries, including those of Vietnam veterans. And as figure 7.3 illustrates, teenage girls, who are more likely to have premature babies and other complications stemming from pregnancy, become pregnant almost twice as often in the United States as in Canada and give birth nearly two and one-quarter times as often.[21]

FIGURE 7-3

Pregnancy, Childbearing and Abortions among Girls Ages 15-19
(per 1,000)

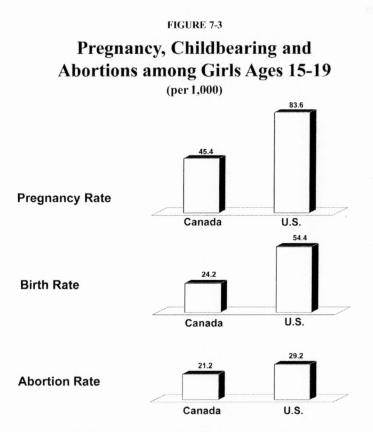

Source: Susheela Singh and Jacqueline E. Darroch, "Adolescent Pregnancy and Childbearing: Levels and Trends in Developed Countries," Alan Guttmacher Institute, *Family Planning Perspectives*, January/February 2000.

NOTES

1. For a discussion of the problems associated with international comparisons of health care spending, see Adrian Towse and Jon Sussex, "'Getting UK Health Care Expenditure Up to the European Union Mean'—What Does That Mean?" *British Medical Journal* vol. 320, no. 7325 (March 4, 2000): 640–42; and Panos Kanavos and Elias Mossialos, "The Methodology of International Comparisons of Health Care Expenditures: Any Lessons for Health Policy?" London School of Economics and Political Science, LSE Health, Discussion Paper No. 3, April 1996, available at www.lse.ac.uk/Depts/lsehsc/papers/Discussion_Papers/dp3.pdf.

2. Pedro P. Barros, "The Black Box of Health Care Expenditure Growth Determinants," *Health Economics* 7, no. 6 (September 1, 1998): 533–44. Of two countries with the same GDP, the country with the faster-growing economy will likely have the higher expenditure. See R. Mark Wilson, "Medical Care Expenditures and GDP Growth in OECD Nations," *American Association of Behavioral and Social Sciences Journal* 2 (Fall 1999): 159–71.

3. Joseph Newhouse, "Medical Care Expenditure: A Cross-National Survey," *Journal of Human Resources* 12 (1977): 115–25; and Joseph Newhouse et al., "Some Interim Results from a Controlled Trial of Cost-Sharing in Health Insurance," *New England Journal of Medicine* (December 17, 1981) 305(25), 1501–1507.

4. Kanavos and Mossialos, "The Methodology of International Comparisons."

5. "OECD Health Systems: Facts and Trends 1960–1991," Organization for Economic Cooperation and Development, 1993.

6. Towse and Sussex, "Getting UK Health Care Expenditure Up."

7. Martin Hensher, Nigel Edwards and Rachel Stokes, "The Hospital of the Future: International Trends in the Provision and Utilization of Hospital Care," *British Medical Journal* vol. 319, no. 7213 (September 25, 1999): 845–48.

8. Gerard F. Anderson, Uwe E. Reinhardt, Peter S. Hussey, and Varduhi Petrosyan, "It's the Prices, Stupid: Why the United States Is So Different From Other Countries," *Health Affairs* 22, no. 3 (May/June 2003): 97, Exhibit 5.

9. Mark V. Pauly, "U.S. Health Care Costs: The Untold True Story," *Health Affairs* 12, no. 3 (Fall 1993): 152–59; and Kanavos and Mossialos, "The Methodology of International Comparisons."

10. Gerard F. Anderson et. al., "Health Spending. and Outcomes: Trends in OECD Countries, 1960–1998," *Health Affairs* (May/June 2000): 150–57.

11. Anderson and Hussey, *Multinational Comparisons of Health Systems Data*.

12. Uwe Reinhardt, Peter S. Hussey and Gerard F. Anderson, "Cross-National Comparisons of Health Systems Using OECD Data, 1999," Health Affairs 21, no. 3, May/June 2002, 169–81.

13. Gwen Gray, "Access to Medical Care Under Strain: New Pressures in Canada Amend Australia," *Journal of Health Politics, Policy and Law* 23, no. 6 (December 1998): 905–47.

14. Gray, "Access to Medical Care."

15. The number of acute care beds per thousand stood at 3.3 in 1999. See Anderson et al., "It's the Prices, Stupid." Canada's acting director of health insurance said

the government was aiming to bring the ration down to two beds per thousand. See Suzanne Rene Possehl, "Northern Plights," *Hospitals & Health Networks* 71, no. 17 (September 5, 1997): 56–60.

16. David Spurgeon, "Canadians Need to Spend C$5bn More a Year on Health Care," *British Medical Journal* 325, no. 7372 (November 9, 2002), 1058.

17. Spurgeon, "Canadians Need to Spend."

18. Jacques Krasny and Ian R. Ferrier, "A Closer Look at Health Care in Canada," *Health Affairs* vol. 10, no. 2 (Summer 1991): 152–58. For a critique of this approach see Daniel R. Waldo and Sally T. Sonnefeld, "U.S./Canadian Health Spending: Methods and Assumptions," *Health Affairs* vol. 10, no. 2 (Summer 1991): 159–164.

19. Waldo and Sonnefeld, "U.S./Canadian Health Spending."

20. Don B. Kates, "Guns and Public Health: Epidemic of Violence or Pandemic of Propaganda?" *Tennessee Law Review* 61 (1994): 513–96.

21. Susheela Singh and Jacqueline E. Darroch, "Adolescent Pregnancy and Childbearing: Levels and Trends in Developed Countries," Alan Guttmacher Institute, *Family Planning Perspectives* 32, no. 1 (January/February 2000), 14–23.

Chapter Eight

Efficiency

MYTH NO. 8: COUNTRIES WITH SINGLE-PAYER NATIONAL HEALTH INSURANCE HOLD DOWN COSTS BY OPERATING MORE EFFICIENT HEALTH CARE SYSTEMS

Advocates of single-payer health insurance often point to the low level of health care spending in countries with national health insurance as evidence of efficient management. But cheap is not the same as efficient. By and large, countries that have slowed the growth of health care spending have done so by *denying services*, not by using resources more efficiently. In Britain, it is not unusual to find a modern laboratory and an antiquated radiology department in the same hospital. Nor is it unusual to find one hospital with a bed shortage near another with a bed surplus. Excellence is random and is often the result of the energy and enthusiasm of a few isolated individuals rather than decisions by hospital management.

How much does it cost a hospital to perform an appendectomy? Outside the United States, it is doubtful that any public hospital could provide the answer. Nor do government-run hospitals typically keep records that would allow anyone else to find out.[1] In organizational skills and managerial efficiency, the public hospitals of other countries lag far behind hospitals in the United States. Nor is it easy for other countries to change course. One reason is that health care is political. Health economist Alain Enthoven has observed that because health care in Britain is so politicized, "it is more difficult to close an unneeded [British] hospital than an unneeded American military base."[2]

INEFFICIENCY IN BRITAIN

Britain has about 20 percent fewer inpatient hospital beds per capita than the United States and about 44 percent fewer than the OECD median of 4.3 per 1,000 population.[3] Partly due to this smaller capacity, it has experienced a persistent shortage of hospital beds. In recent years, the shortage has become critical. Britain also suffers from staffing shortages and is therefore unable to utilize all available beds. Furthermore, beds are often utilized inappropriately. For example, in 2000, 90 percent of hospital geriatric beds were occupied, whereas only 60 percent of maternity beds were occupied. Had the 40 percent of vacant maternity beds been converted to geriatric use, queues for hospital admission would have been much shorter.[4]

On the other hand, long-term care patients who should be in nursing homes, geriatric wards or at home are often found occupying acute care beds in Britain, a practice known as "bed blocking." As a result, many patients must wait for admission and treatment because patients treated earlier are waiting for discharge to an appropriate facility and thus "blocking" access to a bed. Officials estimate that about 3.3 percent of beds are blocked at any given time.[5] And many public health officials think the actual number may be far higher. Liam Fox, the Conservative party's shadow health secretary in the British parliament, has estimated that the true number of blocked beds is closer to 15 percent.[6]

Nicola Sturgeon, a member of the Scottish parliament, reported that 10 percent of acute care beds in Scotland are "occupied by geriatric patients needing residential care."[7] A survey of a hospital in Coventry found that three-fourths of patients occupying beds no longer needed acute care, but had nowhere suitable to go.[8] The problem is so severe that in an attempt to free up more hospital beds for acute care patients, the Department of Health launched a pilot project that sends patients to recover at bed-and-breakfast inns in the countryside.[9]

The statistics on bed utilization indicate bed management in Britain is highly inefficient. More than one million people are waiting for medical treatment in British hospitals at any one time and an estimated 500,000 surgeries were cancelled in the past five years due to the shortage of NHS hospital beds.[10] Yet close to 30,000 beds (16 percent of the total) are empty on any given day.[11] Add to that the number of beds filled with patients who do not belong in a hospital at all and this implies that one out of every three NHS hospital beds are unavailable for acute care patients!

Britain also experiences wide differences in the cost of services within the NHS. Although in general real hospital costs for various procedures are difficult or impossible to determine, one study estimated that costs vary by as much as 58 percent between Britain's most- and least-expensive hospitals. For example[12]:

- The cost of a hip replacement varied from $2,616 to $9,264, a difference of 254 percent.
- The cost of a vasectomy ranged from $211 to over $1,427, a difference of 550 percent.

The cheapest hospital trust in England costs 30 percent below the national average, while the most expensive had costs 60 percent above the average.[13]

INEFFICIENCY IN CANADA

In Canada a large percentage of acute care hospital beds also are used for patients who do not need acute care. The Manitoba Center for Health Policy found that across the provinces from 7 percent to 51 percent of Canadian adult admissions and from 27 percent to 59 percent of the days patients spent in hospitals were for conditions that did not require acute care, although most did need some form of supervised care.[14] Among the findings,

- In Manitoba, 23 percent of the bed days spent by short-stay patients in acute care hospitals were unnecessary.[15]
- In Winnipeg, Manitoba, 40 percent of the acute care beds were used by only a few patients, each staying more than thirty days.[16]

Although the less efficient use of acute care beds generally is attributed to a lack of other facilities, especially for patients needing long-term care, global budgets create incentives to keep chronic patients in acute hospital beds. Hospital managers find it less expensive when a bed is occupied by a long-term patient who needs mostly "hotel" services than when the bed is occupied by a patient who needs more costly treatment.[17] The practice may also make life more convenient for doctors, despite the social cost. Some physicians find it easier and faster to arrange a diagnostic test like a CT scan or stress test for an inpatient and easier to locate the results because they are on the patient's chart.[18]

EFFICIENCY MEASURE: HOSPITAL LENGTH OF STAY

One widely used measure of hospital efficiency is average length of stay (LOS).[19] Hospital-related services are the largest component of health care costs in most countries.[20] Thus, the inappropriate use of hospital facilities has a significant impact on the efficiency of the health care system. It is an inefficient use of resources to fill an acute care hospital bed with a patient awaiting nonemergency care, or a geriatric patient awaiting transfer to a nonacute facility, or simply because the hospital has not gotten around to discharging that patient. This is especially true when there are lengthy waiting lists for hospital admission. Generally, the more efficient the hospital, the more quickly it will admit and discharge patients.[21]

By this standard, U.S. hospitals are ahead of their international counterparts (see figure 8.1).[22] The average length of a hospital stay in the United States is 5.9 days compared to 6.2 days in Australia, 9.0 in the Netherlands, and 9.6 in Germany. Whereas patients from other countries routinely convalesce in a hospital, American patients are more likely to recover at home.

FIGURE 8-1

Average Length of Hospital Stay

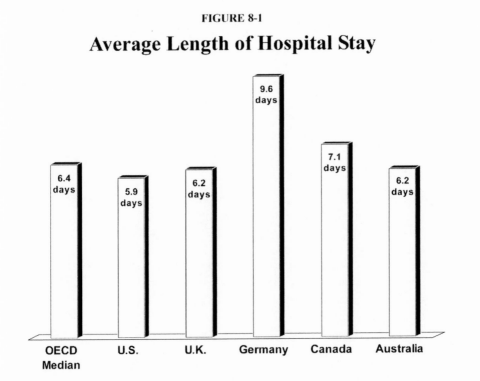

Source: Gerard F. Anderson, Uwe E. Reinhardt, Peter S. Hussey and Varduhi
          Petrosyan, "It's the Prices, Stupid: Why the United States is So Different
          from Other Countries," *Health Affairs*, Vol. 22, No. 3, May/June 2003,
          Exhibit 5: 97.

COST COMPARISON: BRITAIN'S NHS VERSUS U.S. HMOS

A comparison of the NHS and Kaiser Permanente, a large U.S. HMO, concluded that the per capita costs of the two systems were similar. However, the analysis found that Kaiser provided its members with more comprehensive and convenient primary care services and much more rapid access to specialists and hospital admissions. After adjustments for differences between countries, the NHS cost was calculated at $1,764 per capita compared to a Kaiser cost of $1,951.[23] However, figure 8.2 shows the following:

- Kaiser had two and one-half times as many pediatricians, twice as many obstetricians-gynecologists and three times as many cardiologists per enrollee as the NHS.

FIGURE 8-2

Kaiser California vs. NHS
Specialists per 100,000 People

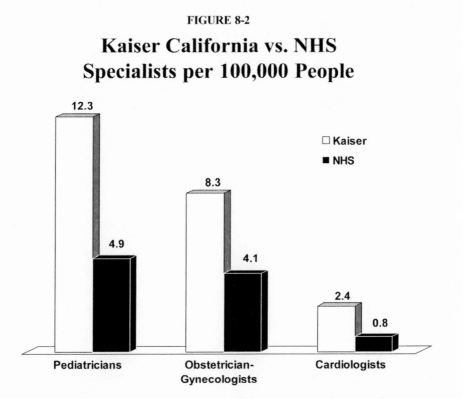

Source: Richard G. A. Feachem, Neelam K. Sekhri and Karen L. White, "Getting More for Their Dollar: A Comparison of the NHS with California's Kaiser Permanente," *British Medical Journal*, January 19, 2002.

- After referral, waiting times to see a specialist were more than six times as long in the NHS.
- For nonemergency hospital admission, 90 percent of Kaiser patients waited less than three months; one-third of NHS patients waited more than five months.

One of the most striking differences between the two health systems was the length of stay. Kaiser had 270 acute care bed days per 1,000 population, whereas NHS patients stayed in the hospital more than three times as long— an average of 1,000 acute care bed days per 1,000 population.[24] In summary, the study found that[25]

> The widely held beliefs that the NHS is efficient and that poor performance in certain areas is largely explained by underinvestment are not supported by this analysis. Kaiser achieved better performance at roughly the same cost as the NHS because of integration throughout the system, efficient management of hospital use, the benefits of competition and greater investment in information technology.

PRIVATE SOLUTIONS FOR THE PROBLEMS OF NATIONAL HEALTH INSURANCE

Several European countries with single-payer health care systems have discovered the value of competition, albeit sometimes reluctantly. European Union regulations that force reductions in taxes have driven some countries to experiment with "internal markets" that introduce private health care providers into the publicly financed system. One example is in Stockholm, the capital of Europe's most heavily socialized welfare state. After first allowing competition by contractors for nonmedical services, the city's Health Services Council began privatizing all primary care in 1998 and sold St. Göran's, one of Sweden's largest hospitals, to a private company in 1999. Most of the funding still comes from the government, which is getting far more for its money than before. A study of the privatization program found[26]

- The cost per consultation in private practices compared to public hospital outpatient clinics ranges from 13 percent lower in general surgery, internal medicine and dermatology to 17 percent lower among ear, nose and throat specialists and 28 percent lower in ophthalmology.
- At St. Göran's, costs for lab and X-ray services fell by 50 percent and overall costs by 30 percent.

- Private nursing home costs were 30 percent lower.
- On average, St. Göran's now treats 100,000 more patients each year than it did as a public hospital, while using fewer resources.

As a result of the experiment, the Health Services Council plans to turn over operations of the seven remaining public acute care hospitals in Stockholm to private investors.

NOTES

1. For Britain, see the discussion in Alain C. Enthoven, "Internal Market Reform of the British Health Service," *Health Affairs* 10, no. 3 (Fall 1991): 60–70. A Canadian observer reports that "Ontario hospitals lag at least a decade behind their U.S. counterparts in expenditure tracking and management information systems." See C. David Naylor, "A Different View of Queues in Ontario," *Health Affairs* 10, no. 3 (Fall 1991): 112.

2. Enthoven, "Internal Market Reform," 62.

3. Gerard Anderson and Peter Sotir Hussey, "Comparing Health System Performance in OECD Countries," *Health Affairs* 20, no. 3 (May/June 2001): 219–32.

4. "Publication of Latest Statistics on Bed Availability and Occupancy for England, 2000–2001."

5. For example, a BBC report claimed that on any given day, around 6,000 (out of a total 186,000 hospital beds) are occupied by "bed blockers." Two-thirds of these are elderly patients in need of less-expensive community facilities. See Karen Allen, "Analysis: How to Beat NHS Gridlock" *BBC News,* October 10, 2001 and "Bed-Blocking a Massive Problem," *BBC News,* April 17, 2002.

6. See Jenny Booth, "Scandal of Stranded Hospital Pensioners: Labour Accused over the Shortage of Money and Nursing Home Places That Leaves Patients Blocking NHS Beds, Reports Jenny Booth," *Sunday Telegraph* (London), August 12, 2001.

7. *Scottish Parliament Official Report* 9, no. 2 (November 16, 2000).

8. Karen Hambridge, "Shocking Truth behind Lack of Hospital Beds: Wards Full of Patients Who Shouldn't Be There," *Coventry Evening Telegraph*, June 30, 2001.

9. See Valerie Elliott, "'Bed Blockers' Farmed Out for B&B Recovery," *The Times* (London), February 9, 2002.

10. Elliott, "'Bed Blockers' Farmed Out."

11. The U.S. occupancy rate of approximately 65 percent is far below Britain's rate of 84 percent. For information on Britain's bed occupancy rate, see "Publication of Latest Statistics on Bed Availability and Occupancy for England, 2000–2001," UK Department of Health Press Release, September 19, 2001.

12. Linda Beecham, "Cost of NHS Operations Varies Widely," *British Medical Journal* vol. 317, no. 7169 (November 14, 1998), 1393.

13. Beecham, "Cost of NHS Operations."

14. Carolyn DeCoster, Sandra Peterson and Paul Kasian, "Alternatives to Acute Care," Manitoba Centre for Health Policy and Evaluation, July 1996.

15. Sharon Bruce et al., "Acuity of Patients Hospitalized for Medical Conditions at Winnipeg Acute Care Hospitals," Manitoba Centre for Health Policy and Evaluation, June 2001.

16. Carolyn DeCoster and Anita Kozyrskyj, "Long-Stay Patients in Winnipeg Acute Care Hospitals," Manitoba Centre for Health Policy and Evaluation, September 2000.

17. Raisa Deber, a professor of health policy at the University of Toronto, described the incentive: "Since hospitals have budgets to follow, they may have to ration the use of expensive procedures even though this might result in waiting lists." Raisa Deber, "Canada's Healthcare System," presentation to the Maine Development Foundation, 2000.

18. DeCoster, Peterson and Kasian, "Alternatives to Acute Care."

19. See, for example, "The New NHS, Modern and Dependable: A National Framework for Assessing Performance," UK Department of Health, 1998, Attachment A.iv and Attachment B.xviii, available at www.doh.gov.uk/newnhs/consdoc/info.htm; Harald Buhaug, "Length of Stay in General Hospitals," available at www.valm.lv/orahs99/Abstr24.html; and Marni D. Brownell and Noralou P. Roos, "Variation in Length of Stay as a Measure of Efficiency in Manitoba Hospitals," *Canadian Medical Association Journal* 152, no. 5 (March 1, 1995): 675–82.

20. In the United States, hospitalization accounts for 42.2 percent of health costs.

21. The actuarial firm Milliman & Robertson has devised the "Length of Stay Efficiency Index," which compares average length of stay by diagnosis-related group (DRG) code and other factors; see www.hospitalefficiencybenchmarks.com. For a discussion of length of stay, see Helen Lippman, "The Bottom Line on Length of Stay," *Business and Health* (April 2001).

22. Gerard F. Anderson, Uwe E. Reinhardt, Peter S. Hussey, and Varduhi Petrosyan, "It's the Prices, Stupid: Why the United States Is So Different from Other Countries," *Health Affairs* 22, no. 3 (May/June 2003).

23. Richard G. A. Feachem, Neelam K. Sekhri and Karen L. White, "Getting More for Their Dollar: A Comparison of the NHS with California's Kaiser Permanente," *British Medical Journal* vol. 324, no. 7330 (January 19, 2002): 135–43.

24. Feachem et al., "Getting More for Their Dollar," 143. The authors noted, "There is ample evidence that reduced length of hospital stay does no harm and, in view of the risk of staying in hospital, may be beneficial."

25. Feachem et al., "Getting More for Their Dollar," 143.

26. A. Wess Mitchell, "Sweden Edges toward Free-Market Medicine," National Center for Policy Analysis, Brief Analysis No. 369, August 31, 2001.

Chapter Nine

Unnecessary Care

MYTH NO. 9: COUNTRIES WITH
SINGLE-PAYER NATIONAL HEALTH CARE
SYSTEMS ELIMINATE UNNECESSARY MEDICAL CARE

A frequent criticism of the U.S. health care system is that it is wasteful because a considerable number of procedures are "unnecessary." For example, in 1989 Robert Brook of the Rand Corporation asserted that "perhaps one-fourth of hospital days, one-fourth of procedures and two-fifths of medications could be done without."[1] To support this contention, Rand researchers pointed to wide variations in 123 medical procedures for Medicare patients in various parts of the country.[2] The rate at which the procedures were performed varied by as much as six, seven, or eight to one, with no apparent explanation. Areas that were high in performing one procedure were often low in performing another. Other studies have found similar results.[3] But knowing there are variations does not reveal whether some patients are being shortchanged and others overtreated.[4]

THE RAND STUDY OF UNNECESSARY CARE

A subsequent Rand study collected medical records for 5,000 Medicare patients treated in 1981 and convened a panel of experts to judge the appropriateness of three procedures.[5] The results showed that in slightly more than a fifth of the cases, the procedure performed was judged inappropriate and therefore unnecessary. For carotid endarterectomy (the removal of plaque in major arteries to the brain), the procedure was judged appropriate only about one-third of the time.[6] National media widely reported these results, and they

93

became Exhibit A in building the case for the managed care revolution during the 1990s (see table 9.1). But a closer examination reveals more than first meets the eye. For example, why did Rand need to convene a panel of experts? Because researchers could not answer questions about appropriateness by merely consulting the medical literature. And the convened experts were far less unified than media reports suggested.

REEXAMINING THE EVIDENCE OF UNNECESSARY CARE

The classifications depicted in table 9.1 were decided by a majority vote. Table 9.2 presents a different way of looking at the Rand study, showing the number of times that seven of nine experts agreed. (The two opinions ignored are the two most extreme.) As the table shows, seven of the nine found only 12 percent of the procedures to be inappropriate, not 22 percent. And even this degree of consensus is misleading. In the Rand study, each expert initially expressed a personal judgment. Then they met for discussions in which group pressure favored consensus and members often changed their minds.[7] Indeed, the most remarkable fact about the Rand study was that despite their efforts to arrive at a definitive judgment, seven of nine experts could agree less than half the time that the procedures were either definitely appropriate or definitely inappropriate.

EVIDENCE TODAY

What inferences can we draw from a study of medical records in 1981 for the practice of medicine today? Since then, major changes have been made in the way hospitals are run. For better or for worse, American physicians are now more closely scrutinized by peers and third-party payers than physicians anywhere else in the world. This scrutiny, coupled with the prospect of malpractice liability lawsuits, limits the likelihood of procedures that do more harm than good. It still may happen in HMOs as well as fee-for-service insurance plans, but it is much less likely than two decades ago. The results of three studies of surgery in New York State in 1990 are consistent with this judgment. In all three cases, the fraction of inappropriate procedures was judged to be 4 percent or less.[8]

MEDICAL ART VERSUS MEDICAL SCIENCE

Medical science has clearly advanced over the past two decades. Despite that fact, practicing physicians still hold widely differing opinions about the appropriateness of care.

TABLE 9-1

Rand Corporation Study on Unnecesary Medicine as Reported by the U.S. National Media

	Panel's Assessment[1]		
	Appropriate	Equivocal	Inappropriate
Coronary angiography[2]	74%	9%	17%
Carotid endarterectomy[3]	35%	32%	32%
Upper gastrointestinal endoscopy[4]	72%	11%	17%
Overall	60%	18%	22%

[1] Based on medical records of 5,000 Medicare patients.

[2] Use of X-rays and dye to expose obstructions of the heart.

[3] Surgical removal of obstructions in major arteries to the brain.

[4] Fiber optic examination of the esophagus, stomach and upper intestine.

Source: Rand Corporation study results reported in the *Wall Street Journal*, March 22, 1990.

More than half the procedures in the Rand study fell between the do-no-harm standard and the conservative standard of performing a procedure only if it is definitely appropriate (see table 9.1). In the New York studies, the "uncertain" range was as high as 38 percent. These findings imply an enormous range over which discretion can be exercised and still fall within the bounds

TABLE 9-2

More Details on the Rand Study

	Percent of Time 7 to 9 Experts Agree that Procedure Is:	
	Appropriate	Inappropriate
Coronary angiography	50%	12%
Carotid endarterectomy	13%	17%
Upper gastrointestinal endoscopy	46%	7%
Overall	36%	12%

Source: Robert H. Brook, "Practice Guidelines and Practicing Medicine: Are They Compatible?" *Journal of the American Medical Association*, December 1, 1989.

of good science and medical ethics. They also imply that often there is no objective "right" answer and that the practice of medicine remains as much an
art as a science. Thus, the debate about unnecessary or inappropriate treatments is far from over.[9] Put crudely, these studies point to the prospect of a
health plan being able to make a great deal of money by substantially reducing the number of procedures performed without violating any professional
code of conduct.

THE FIND-NO-HARM APPROACH
TO IDENTIFYING INEFFICIENT CARE

Researchers at Milliman & Robertson (M&R), a leading actuarial consulting
firm, have taken a different approach to this issue. Rather than attempt to determine whether procedures are appropriate, M&R analysts sought to determine whether fewer days in a hospital can cause detectable harm. If they
could detect none, M&R concluded that the extra days represented unnecessary (read: inefficient) care.[10]

For example, take groups of similar patients hospitalized for two, four and
six days for a specific condition. Suppose medical records show that the
health outcomes of patients with a two-day hospital stay are no different from
those of patients with four- or six-day stays. M&R would conclude that the
four-day stay involved two days and the six-day stay four days of unnecessary hospitalization. Using a similar methodology, suppose people treated as
outpatients fared just as well as people hospitalized for the same condition.
Then M&R would conclude that all the inpatient days were unnecessary. Pro-
ceeding in this way, M&R estimated the total number of unnecessary hospital days for the country as a whole. Table 9.3 shows the following:[11]

- M&R estimated that two-thirds of hospital days of nonelderly patients were
  unnecessary in Newark, Philadelphia, Pittsburgh and New Orleans.
- The range was from 35 percent in Portland to 72 percent in New York City.
- Nationwide, M&R estimated that 54 percent of all inpatient days were unnecessary.[12]

For the elderly (Medicare) population, M&R estimated that 53 percent of
inpatient care was unnecessary, ranging from 34 percent in Honolulu to 65
percent in New York City.

Two critical assumptions lie behind these estimates. First, in deciding
whether hospital stays were unnecessary, M&R looked only at outcomes and
not at risk reduction. For example, even if the four-day hospital stay produced

TABLE 9-3

Milliman & Robertson Estimate
of Unnecessary Days in U.S. Hospitals
(Nonelderly Population)

Market	Estimated Percentage of Days Unnecessary
New York	72%
New Orleans	68%
Pittsburgh	67%
Philadelphia	67%
Newark	67%
National average	54%
Seattle	41%
San Diego	40%
Salt Lake City	39%
Phoenix	38%
Portland	35%

)urces: David V. Axene, Richard L. Doyle and Dirk van der Burch, *Research Report: Analysis of Medically Unnecessary Inpatient Services* (Seattle: Milliman & Robertson, 1997); and Milliman & Robertson, *Length of Stay Efficiency Index for 1996* (Seattle: Milliman & Robertson, 1997).

the same medical outcome as the two-day stay, the risks to which patients were exposed were different. On the one hand, simply being in a hospital adds to risk. According to one study, two million Americans pick up infections during a stay in the hospital each year—almost 10 infections for every 1,000 patient days—and 106,000 of these were fatal. Moreover, one of every 300 patients dies of adverse drug reaction, making that one of the leading causes of death.[13] Although these results have been disputed, no one thinks the risks are negligible.[14] But being in a hospital reduces risk in other ways. If the patient's health worsens, the hospital can bring highly specialized resources to bear right away.

Other things being equal the less time spent in the hospital, the better. But not everyone shares this view. Take well-baby delivery, for example. Managed care organizations have decided that two nights in a hospital and perhaps even one night is unnecessary. But one study found that babies released from the hospital less than seventy-two hours after birth have a small increased risk of readmission.[15]

A second assumption is that because a length-of-stay objective is met somewhere in the United States, it can be met everywhere. M&R encouraged this interpretation by publishing guidelines on appropriate lengths of stay for surgical procedures.[16] HMOs and other managed care organizations used the guidelines to pressure providers. Physicians were appalled. The reason? M&R's recommended lengths of stay are very different from what most physicians think is appropriate for their patients.[17]

- Whereas M&R recommended that women stay in a hospital a little over one day for a normal baby delivery and two and one-half days for a cesarean, the national average is more than two days for the former and more than four for the latter.
- Whereas M&R recommended that mastectomies be done on an outpatient basis, the average length of stay for the country as a whole is two and one-half days.
- In the case of the high-risk procedure of esophagectomy (removal of the esophagus), M&R recommended five days compared to an average actual patient stay of thirteen days.
- For a mid-shaft femur fracture (broken thigh bone), M&R recommended one day, while the average patient stay is six days.
- For craniotomy (brain surgery), the difference is five days and for a radical hysterectomy, seven days.

Clearly, what M&R recommended is not what most doctors might prescribe. And the use of such guidelines to press for premature patient releases has caused political turmoil. For example, in response to patient complaints about drive-through deliveries, a 1997 federal law guarantees mothers the right to hospital stays of two days for well-baby delivery and four days for a cesarean. Dozens of states have passed similar laws. Who is right: M&R, the doctors or the politicians? In some cases M&R may simply be wrong. In other cases, M&R may theoretically be right, but its guidelines cannot be met through the simple expedient of early release. As the following case study notes, meeting the guidelines may require completely changing the way doctors practice medicine.

CASE STUDY: MASTECTOMIES

M&R guidelines state that an ordinary mastectomy can be performed on an outpatient with a stay as short as six hours. There is a facility that meets this standard, but it is the only place in the country that does so—the Johns Hopkins Breast Center. Under the leadership of William Dooley and Lillie Shockney, the center has revolutionized breast surgery by investing time, effort and energy in learning how to do the procedure differently from standard practice.

For example, whereas a mastectomy would ordinarily average about two hours, Dooley does it in forty-seven minutes. Because the center uses a different anesthesia and anesthetizes the patient for much less time, recovery is quicker and side effects are fewer. Patients have the option of spending the night in the hospital, but most choose to go home. They can do so because several days prior to surgery they go through a three-hour training session with their care partner (usually someone who lives in the home with the patient). Such training is important, because patients need to be able to monitor their own progress and recognize signs of potential trouble. In addition, after surgery a nurse visits the patients in their homes twice.

The result is lower cost, higher quality and satisfied patients. Yet, if an HMO insisted on outpatient surgery without changes in hospital technique and patient training, the risk of unhappy patients reappearing in the emergency room with further complications might greatly increase.[18]

ECONOMIC IMPLICATIONS OF THE M&R AND RAND STUDIES

What the Johns Hopkins Breast Center has designed is a more efficient way to perform breast surgery. Women are not simply sent home earlier; they are enabled to go home early. And the fact that more hospitals around the country have not copied the technique indicates how inefficient our health care system is, compared to other markets.

The Rand study focused on the decision to perform surgery and strongly implied that unnecessary care was being delivered for economic reasons. However, the opposite incentive is present with respect to length of stay. Most physicians have a direct or indirect economic incentive to reduce length of stay.[19] The fact that it takes so long for efficient surgical techniques to be widely adopted implies that doctors are not responding quickly enough to economic incentives!

Why not? It is tempting to conclude that physicians find it easier to continue inefficient surgical procedures and the risks of early release than to invest in learning more efficient techniques. Unfortunately, this conclusion is consistent with the idea that managed care rewards cost reduction at the expense of quality more than cost reduction produced by greater efficiency and subsequent quality improvement.

UNNECESSARY CARE IN OTHER COUNTRIES

One might suppose that in countries where health care is rationed and many medical needs go unmet, doctors would tend to provide only "necessary" care. This is not the case. According to Rand research, those who receive care may not be those most in need of care. A review of the medical records on coronary artery bypass surgery performed in the Trent region of Britain found many were performed for less than appropriate reasons (using both British and American criteria).[20] Overall, Rand researchers found that[21]

- 21 percent of British coronary angiographies and 16 percent of coronary artery bypass graft surgeries were performed for inappropriate reasons.
- In some regions, coronary angiography and coronary artery bypass procedures were found to be inappropriate about 50 percent of the time.
- In the Northwest Thames region, 60 percent of gall bladder removals with a laparoscope were found to be inappropriate.

Despite waiting lists, health authorities appear not to question the appropriateness of the procedures for which patients are waiting.[22] Rand researcher Robert Brook, himself a physician, told a U.S. Senate committee, "I was shocked to find that half of the people who actually got cardiac revascularization did not meet criteria established by physicians in the UK for getting those procedures."[23]

Rand researchers found similar results in other countries with national health insurance. For example:

- In Israel, 29 percent of gall bladder removals were performed for "less-than-appropriate" reasons.[24]
- A panel of reviewers found that 19 percent of referrals of Swedish patients for coronary revascularization were inappropriate.[25]

The Rand summary concluded, "Contrary to the researchers' expectations, habitual rationing of resources did not restrict use of these sophisticated and expensive treatments to only those who would most clearly benefit from them."[26] Other studies have come to similar conclusions.[27]

NOTES

1. Robert H. Brook, "Practice Guidelines and Practicing Medicine: Are They Compatible?" *Journal of the American Medical Association* 262, no. 21 (December

1, 1989), 3028. The Rand Corporation has published a number of studies over the past decade examining the appropriateness of various medical and surgical procedures. For a summary and selected bibliography of Rand research, see "Assessing the Appropriateness of Care," Rand Corporation, Health Research Highlights, RB-4522, 1998. The methodology used in the studies is described by Robert H. Brook, "The Rand/UCLA Appropriateness Method," in K. A. McCormick, S. R. Moore and R. A. Siegel, eds., "Clinical Practice Guidelines Development: Methodology Perspectives," available as Rand Reprint RP-395, 1995.

2. A summary of Rand Corporation research may be found in Mark R. Chassin, ed., *The Appropriateness of Selected Medical and Surgical Procedures* (Ann Arbor, Mich.: Health Administration Press, 1989).

3. See, for example, John E. Wennberg, "Understanding Geographic Variations in Health Care Delivery," *New England Journal of Medicine* 340, no. 1 (January 7, 1999): 52–53.

4. John W. Dawson, "Practice Variations: A Challenge for Physicians," *Journal of the American Medical Association* 258, no. 18 (November 13, 1987), 2570.

5. Mark R. Chassin et al., "Does Inappropriate Use Explain Geographic Variations in the Use of Health Care Services? A Study of Three Procedures," *Journal of the American Medical Association* 258, no. 18 (November 13, 1987): 2533–37; Jacqueline Kosecoff et al., "Obtaining Clinical Data on the Appropriateness of Medical Care in Community Practice," *Journal of the American Medical Association* 258, no. 18 (November 13, 1987): 2538–42; and Mark R. Chassin et al., "How Coronary Angiography Is Used: Clinical Determinants of Appropriateness," *Journal of the American Medical Association* 258, no. 18 (November 13, 1987): 2543–47.

6. "Appropriateness" was not determined by Monday morning quarterbacking, rather it was based on indications prior to the procedure. A procedure was judged appropriate if the expected benefit (increased life expectancy, relief of pain, etc.) exceeded the expected negative consequences (mortality, morbidity, etc.) by a margin sufficient to justify the procedure.

7. "Disagreement among the panelists diminished following their discussions, but by no means disappeared." Chassin, ed., *The Appropriateness of Selected Medical and Surgical Procedures,* 8.

8. Lucian Leape et al., "The Appropriateness of Use of Coronary Artery Bypass Graft Surgery in New York State," *Journal of the American Medical Association* 269, no. 6 (February 10, 1993): 753–60; Lee Hilborne et al., "The Appropriateness of Use of Percutaneous Transluminal Coronary Angioplasty in New York State," *Journal of the American Medical Association* 269, no. 6 (February 10, 1993): 761–65; Steven Bernstein et al., "The Appropriateness of Use of Coronary Angiography in New York State," *Journal of the American Medical Association* 269, no. 6 (February 10, 1993): 766–69.

9. Dawson, "Practice Variations." Also see David H. Mark, "Variations and Inappropriateness Are Not the Same," *Journal of the American Medical Association* 263, no. 23 (June 20, 1990): 3149–50.

10. This is part of M&R's efforts to aid employers and insurers in managing their costs.

11. David V. Axene, Richard L. Doyle and Dirk van der Burch, "Research Report: Analysis of Medically Unnecessary Inpatient Services," Milliman & Robertson, 1997; and "Length of Stay Efficiency Index for 1996," Milliman & Robertson, 1997.

12. M&R's estimate is based upon a population of under-sixty-five, private sector insured patients and excludes a small number of highly efficient managed care patients. Also see Axene, Doyle and van der Burch, "Research Report."

13. Jason Lazarou, Bruce H. Pomeranz and Paul N. Corey, "Incidence of Adverse Drug Reactions in Hospitalized Patients: A Meta-Analysis of Prospective Studies," *Journal of the American Medical Association* 279, no. 15 (April 15, 1995): 1200–5. See also Lawrence K. Altman, "Experts See Need to Control Antibiotics and Hospitals Infections," *New York Times*, March 12, 1998; Barbara Starfield, "Is U.S. Health Care Really the Best in the World?" *Journal of the American Medical Association* 284, no. 4 (July 26, 2000): 483–85, available at http://jama.ama-assn.org/cgi/content/full/284/4/483.

14. See Arthur Allen, "Overreaction," *New Republic* (June 8, 1998): 14–15.

15. The risk is of readmission for hyperbilirubinemia, an elevated level of bilirubin in the blood that can cause jaundice. See M. Jeffrey Maisels and Elizabeth Kring, "Length of Stay, Jaundice, and Hospital Readmission," *Pediatrics* 101, no. 6 (June 1998): 995–98.

16. The length of stay numbers in table VI were taken from the *Bulletin of the American College of Surgeons*, April 1997.

17. Milliman & Robertson, "The Length of Stay Efficiency Index," *Perspectives*, Milliman & Robertson, July 1995, with examples available online at www.op .net/~jcookson/hlos.html; and Robert Rutledge et al., "An Analysis of 25 Milliman & Robertson Guidelines for Surgery," *Annals of Surgery* 228, no. 4 (1998): 579–87.

18. Among fee-for-service patients, about 10 percent of mastectomies without complications are performed as outpatient procedures, with a hospital stay of less than 24 hours. The risk of rehospitalization would be about 3.0 percent to 3.5 percent if all women were treated outpatient. See Joan L. Warren et al., "Trends and Outcomes of Outpatient Mastectomy in Elderly Women," *Journal of the National Cancer Institute* 90, no. 11 (June 3, 1998): 833–40.

19. Almost all physicians under managed care contracts have a direct financial interest in lowering hospitalization costs by reducing the length of stay. Fee-for-service insurance, including Medicare, often pays fixed fees for hospital procedures as well.

20. Steven J. Bernstein et al., "The Appropriateness of the Use of Cardiovascular Procedures: British versus U.S. Perspectives," Rand Corporation, RP-269, 1994.

21. Robert H. Brook, "Appropriateness: The Next Frontier," *British Medical Journal* 308, no. 6923 (January 22, 1994): 218–19. Also see Robert H. Brook et al., "A Method for the Detailed Assessment of the Appropriateness of Medical Technologies," *International Journal of Technology Assessment in Health Care* 2 (1986): 53–63.

22. Harry Hemingway and Bobbie Jacobson, "Queues for Cure?" *British Medical Journal* 310, no. 6983 (April 1, 1995): 818–19.

23. Robert H. Brook, "Ensuring Delivery of Necessary Care in the U.S.," Statement before the U.S. Senate Committee on Health, Education and Labor and Pensions, March 2, 1999. Also see Bernstein et al., "The Appropriateness of the Use of

Cardiovascular Procedures: British Versus U.S. Perspectives," *International Journal of Technology Assessment in Health Care* 9, no. 1 (1993): 3–10.

24. "Assessing the Appropriateness of Care," Rand Corp., RB-4522.

25. Steven J. Bernstein et al., "Appropriateness of Referral of Coronary Angiography Patients in Sweden," *Heart* 81, no. 5 (May 1999): 470–77.

26. "Assessing the Appropriateness of Care," Rand Corp., RB-4522.

27. See Kathryn Fitch et al., "European Criteria for the Appropriateness and Necessity of Coronary Revascularization Procedures," *European Journal of Cardio-Thoracic Surgery* 18, no. 4 (2000): 380–87.

Chapter Ten

Administrative Costs

MYTH NO. 10: A SINGLE-PAYER NATIONAL HEALTH CARE SYSTEM WOULD REDUCE THE ADMINISTRATIVE COSTS OF U.S. HEALTH CARE

Advocates of single-payer health insurance frequently claim that private health insurance is inefficient because of the administrative costs associated with multiple insurance firms. A study by Steffie Woolhandler, a prominent member of the Physicians' Working Group on Single-Payer National Health Insurance, and her colleagues estimates that administrative costs account for close to one-third of U.S. health care expenditures (31.0 percent), nearly twice as much as in Canada (16.7 percent).[1] Based on such studies, the Physicians' Working Group claims that a single-payer health care system would result in large savings by eliminating "the high overhead and profits of the private, investor-owned insurance industry and reducing spending for marketing and other satellite services."[2] However, over a number of years, Woolhandler's estimates of the proportion of health care costs consumed by administration has grown for both Canada and the United States. Either "inefficiency" in the Canadian system is growing at a rate similar to that for health care in the United States — or her definition of administrative costs has changed significantly.[3]

The Congressional Research Service has estimated administrative costs for Medicare at 2 percent of total program costs, compared to 9.5 percent for private insurance and 11.9 percent for HMOs.[4] Many single-payer advocates have used this estimate as an argument for forcing all Americans to join Medicare.

These estimates are misleading, however. Determining the administrative costs of any government program is difficult, if not impossible. And comparisons with the private sector are problematic. Part of the reason is that government regulators can shift administrative costs to physicians or patients, just as tax collectors shift the cost of record keeping and data collection onto taxpayers. For example, a study by the American Medical Association estimated that a physician spends an average of six minutes on every Medicare claim (compared, say, to twenty minutes spent with the patient) and the physician's staff spends an average of one hour.[5]

ADMINISTRATIVE COSTS AND EFFICIENCY

In general, nobody knows how to measure administrative costs. For example, should we count as "administrative" all activities other than doctor-patient contact? What about keeping patient records? What about reviewing patient records? What about reviews of doctor behavior to make sure patients are not being abused and are receiving appropriate care? What about reviews of prescriptions in an effort to lower the rate of adverse drug reactions? What about paperwork and other procedures instituted to ensure appropriate use of MRI scans? Answers to all of these questions require subjective judgments.

A more basic objection is that minimizing administrative costs should not be our goal. Conventional wisdom holds that the less a health care system spends on administration, the more efficient it must be. Yet, the administrative costs of any health care system could be reduced by firing all of the administrators and abolishing all reporting requirements. Most systems would perform far less efficiently as a result. The real goal is not to get administrative costs as low as possible, but to make the overall system perform as efficiently as possible. To accurately measure the net cost (or gain) to society from administrative procedures, one has to compare the costs with the benefits they produce.

A similar observation holds for marketing and other costs of competition. Money could be saved, for example, by abolishing all car dealerships and advertising by auto producers. Additional money could also be saved by eliminating competition among different automakers (producing numerous models) by building a single model of automobile. Sally Pipes and Michael Lynch of the Pacific Research Institute put it like this:

> Most likely, administrative costs—marketing, selling and invoicing—were a lot lower for the East German Trabant than for a Honda or a Ford. But it does not logically follow that the Trabant is superior. Indeed, the opposite is the case. Multiple payers, or producers, whether in cars, housing, food, clothing or health care, produce product differentiation and spur competition that promotes the production of excellence. In the health care sector, multiple payers provide personalized health care options for U.S. citizens.[6]

We could simply pay taxes and have government provide us with a new automobile every few years. But the end result would be decreased efficiency and less consumer satisfaction, both of which are characteristic of socialist systems. If socialism worked, the economies of communist countries would not have collapsed.

MONOPOLY VERSUS COMPETITION

Regardless of how administrative costs are measured, an article of faith among single-payer advocates is that one insurer paying all bills is better than several insurers competing against each other. But is that really true? To test the assumption, consider the one group of Americans who have no choice of primary insurer: senior citizens on Medicare. Despite its political popularity, Medicare violates almost all of the principles of sound insurance. It pays too many small bills the elderly could easily afford themselves while leaving them exposed to thousands of dollars of potential out-of-pocket expenses, including drug costs. For instance, each year about 750,000 Medicare beneficiaries spend more than $5,000 out of pocket.[7]

To prevent financial devastation from these medical expenses, about two-thirds of Medicare beneficiaries acquire supplemental insurance through a former employer or direct purchase. However, most of these "Medigap" policies do not cover prescriptions and coverage is often incomplete among those that do. Moreover, having a second health plan to fill the holes in the first is wasteful. Seniors with Medigap insurance spend 30 percent more on health care than those without it.[8] To make matters worse, Congress recently passed legislation that will create another optional benefit, covering prescription drugs. Many seniors will soon be paying three premiums to three plans, with all the waste and inefficiency that implies.

As we shall see in chapter 18, dollar for dollar, drugs offer a better return on health care spending than other major therapies.[9] Yet Medicare's practice of covering very few prescription drugs encourages doctors and their patients to choose physician and hospital services instead of less costly, more appropriate drug therapies. Ironically, Medicare will pay to treat a stroke victim in a hospital, but will not pay for the drugs that might have prevented the stroke in the first place.

Medicare's benefit structure has failed to keep pace with modern medicine in other ways. Medicare will pay to amputate the leg of a diabetic, but not for the chronic care that could have made the amputation unnecessary. About 28 percent of all Medicare spending is for patients in the last year of life.[10] Yet, while spending billions on patients who are about to die, Medicare will not pay for the common sense care that would prevent many premature deaths.

Why is the Medicare program so bad? The answer is politics. Almost forty years ago, when Congress created Medicare, the insurance was quite adequate. In designing Medicare, Congress simply copied the standard Blue Cross plan of the day, in part to placate special interest pressures from doctor and hospital organizations. Through the years, medical science has changed, medical economics has changed, and private insurance has changed. But Medicare has not.[11] Once a huge spending program is in place, vested interest constituencies form around every part of it. Whereas private insurance can change and adapt to market conditions at the drop of a hat, even minor changes in Medicare take years.[12]

ADMINISTRATIVE COSTS OF PRIVATE INSURANCE

In general, critics have overestimated the size of private sector administrative costs and underestimated the benefits. The presence of multiple payers in the U.S. system reflects different tastes and preferences among consumers for such amenities as varied levels of copayment, choice of physician network, limited waiting for physician visits, and so forth. Additionally, all private health insurance companies use a portion of a policyholder's premium to assure the remaining funds are spent wisely, while providing quick and convenient service. In doing so, American health plans control moral hazard (the tendency to overconsume when the service is perceived as being free), rather than relying on waiting lines to ration services. Americans pay for the ability to receive medical services when needed rather than having to wait for treatment.

ADMINISTRATIVE COSTS OF PUBLIC PROGRAMS

As noted, a number of studies claim to show that the Canadian system is simply better at controlling administrative costs.[13] However, these studies only focus on inputs into administration—administrative salaries, costs of paperwork, and so forth. Health economist Patricia Danzon of the University of Pennsylvania's Wharton School of Business points out that a public insurer essentially performs most of the same functions found in private insurance. It must reimburse providers for services performed, collect "premiums" (usually from taxes) and attempt to control moral hazard (that is, limit utilization).[14] Likewise, public insurers incur overhead costs, but these are often difficult to analyze using traditional cost accounting methods. Government accounting practices invariably underestimate the real cost of government provision of goods and services. The true cost is often hidden in a complex bureaucratic reporting and tracking system. In both Canada and the United States, auditing expenses for health services are usually included in the budgets of other public agencies.

Collecting taxes or lobbying for additional funding are not included in the overhead expense of public programs, whereas collecting premiums and marketing would count toward the cost of a private health insurer.

Cost comparisons also usually ignore the effects of administration on the efficiency of the health care system in meeting consumer needs, says Danzon. One cannot legitimately calculate administrative costs of single-payer health systems without including adverse effects on patients. These include the excessive time patients spend waiting for treatment, lost productivity caused by lack of advanced medical equipment, and reduced quality of life when certain procedures are unavailable. For example, the physician fee structure found in Canada is designed to limit the volume of procedures performed in doctors' offices. As a result, patients are often forced to make multiple visits to get the same services they could receive in one visit.

Actuary Mark Litow (M&R) estimated the hidden costs (inclusive of taxes) in public programs. He found that Medicare and Medicaid spend 26.9 cents for every dollar of benefits, compared to 16.2 cents spent by private insurance (see figure 10.1).[15] Thus, he estimates that government spends 66 percent more than the private sector per dollar of benefits delivered.

FIGURE 10-1

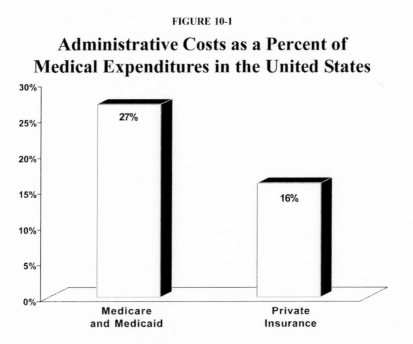

Administrative Costs as a Percent of Medical Expenditures in the United States

Source: Mark Litow and the Technical Committee of the Council for Affordable Health Insurance (CAHI), "Rhetoric vs. Reality: Comparing Public and Private Health Care Administrative Costs," Council for Affordable Health Insurance, March 1994.

GOVERNMENT DISTORTIONS OF PRIVATE INSURANCE

Federal tax policy distorts the health care market by subsidizing health insurance purchased through an employer and penalizing individuals who manage their own health care dollars and pay medical bills directly. Under our tax system, employees (through their employers) can spend unlimited amounts on third-party health insurance, all tax free. At the same time, funds that middle-income employees set aside as self-insurance to pay small medical bills typically face a 25 percent income tax, a 15.3 percent payroll tax (FICA, or Federal Insurance Contributions Act tax) and a 4, 5 or 6 percent state and local income tax.[16] In short, government takes almost half the deposit before it goes into the employees' savings account.

As a result of federal tax policies, most employees are overinsured. They use third parties to pay for routine checkups, diagnostic tests and other small medical bills that could more efficiently be paid out of pocket. Too much insurance encourages people to be wasteful health care consumers. It also adds to administrative costs.[17]

REDUCING ADMINISTRATIVE COSTS
WITH MEDICAL SAVINGS ACCOUNTS

A handful of countries have chosen a different way. In Singapore, workers are required to deposit 6 percent of their salaries each year in personal medical savings accounts (MSAs) called Medisave accounts. When Singapore residents need medical care, they pay the bills from their Medisave funds and avoid many of the administrative burdens of health insurance. They also have catastrophic insurance, which is mainly how they pay hospital bills.[18]

MSAs also exist in South Africa, where they are typically used to pay expenses below the insurance deductible of about $1,200. Since their introduction in 1994, MSA plans have captured about 65 percent of the private insurance market there. These plans have pioneered the use of debit cards to withdraw funds from MSAs to pay for medical services, further reducing administrative costs. Discovery Health, a private insurer, is developing the same type of system for pharmaceutical purchases. Information from a Discovery Health card (and the drug prescribed) is entered into the pharmacy computer. The pharmacy then sends this information electronically to Discovery Health. The insurer checks the patient's MSA balance, verifies drug coverage and any deductible and authorizes payment to the pharmacy.[19]

Dr. David Allen, the Kentucky network medical director for Aetna, estimates that it costs Aetna close to five times more to process a claim submitted on paper than it does a claim submitted electronically.[20] Several companies are experimenting with technology that would put a patient's entire medical record online.[21] This would allow physicians immediate access to each patient's complete medical history. Putting medical records online could be costly. But it might be less costly than the current system under which physicians often treat patients without access to their records and spend far too much of their time dealing with paperwork.[22]

Most medical bills could be paid by patients from health savings accounts (HSAs) with debit cards, relying on third-party insurance to pay only catastrophic expenses.[23] In August of 2003 the U.S. Internal Revenue Service paved the way for the widespread use of debit cards to access personal health accounts.[24] This development is especially important since swiping a debit card across a health care provider's card reader bypasses much of the administrative burden of insurance billing and collecting. It is no coincidence that most of these innovations are occurring in the United States or in countries with less regulated health care systems.

Some patients in the United States already have HSAs of one sort or another. The Health Insurance Portability and Accountability Act (HIPAA) of 1996 created a five-year demonstration for MSAs, but imposed unnecessary restrictions on them.[25] Although 750,000 accounts were allowed by the pilot project, only an estimated 70,000 were actually created.

In a revenue ruling in June 2002, the IRS clarified the use of health reimbursement arrangements (HRAs) under section 105 of the IRS code. Within one year about 1.5 million people were enrolled in these consumer-driven health plans, and such plans are estimated to make up 20 percent of the group market by 2005 and possibly as much as 50 percent by 2007.[26]

The Medicare Prescription Drug and Modernization Act (2003) created HSAs, which have virtually none of the regulatory restrictions of MSAs and which will replace them. In principle, HSAs are available to 250 million (nonelderly) Americans. Like most personal health accounts, they will allow employees to pay directly for medical expenses in conjunction with a high-deductible health plan.[27] Unused funds will roll over from year to year for future use and accumulated balances will be available for medical expenses in retirement.[28]

NOTES

1. Steffie Woolhandler, Terry Campbell and David U. Himmelstein, "Costs of Health Care Administration in the United States and Canada," *New England Journal of Medicine* 349, no. 8 (August 21, 2003): 768–75.

2. See Steffie Woolhandler et al., "Proposal of the Physicians' Working Group for Single-Payer National Health Insurance."

3. See Steffie Woolhandler and David U. Himmelstein, "The Deteriorating Administrative Efficiency of the U.S. Health Care System," *New England Journal of Medicine* 324, no. 18 (May 2, 1991): 1253–58. This study put administrative costs in the U.S. health care system at between 19.3 percent and 24.1 percent of total spending, compared to between 8.4 percent and 11.1 percent of health care spending in Canada. For a critique of the study's methodology by the HIAA, see *Medical Benefits* 8, no. 10 (May 30, 1991): 5. A few years later, they found administrative costs accounted for an average of 26 percent of total U.S. hospital costs. See Steffie Woolhandler and David Himmelstein, "Cost of Care and Administration at For-Profit and Other Hospitals in the United States," *New England Journal of Medicine* 336, no. 11 (March 13, 1997): 769–74.

4. "Administrative Costs: Medicare Compared to Private Insurance and HMOs, 1993," figure 3.29, table 3.29, prepared by the Congressional Research Service, "Medicare and Health Care Chartbook," Ways and Means Committee, U.S. House of Representatives.

5. See the American Medical Association Center for Health Policy Research, "The Administrative Burden of Health Insurance on Physicians," *SMS Report* 3, no. 2 (1989).

6. Sally C. Pipes and Michael Lynch, "False Promise of Single-Payer Health Care: A Close Look Inside the 'California Health Security Act,'" Pacific Research Institute, 1998.

7. U.S Department of Health and Human Services, "Medicare and Medicaid Statistical Supplement, 1999," *Health Care Financial Review*, Publication No. 03417, Centers for Medicare and Medicaid Services, U.S Department of Health and Human Services, November 1999, figure 19, p. 37.

8. Most studies have found that the increased spending is due to perverse insurance incentives and not to worsening health among seniors. For a discussion, see Susan L. Ettner, "Adverse Selection and the Purchase of Medigap Insurance by the Elderly," *Journal of Health Economics* 16, no. 5 (October 1, 1997): 543–62; and Michael D. Hurd and Kathleen McGarry, "Medical Insurance and the Use of Health Care Services by the Elderly," *Journal of Health Economics* 16, no. 2 (April 1997): 129–54. Also see Sandra Christensen and Judy Shinogle, "Effects of Supplemental Coverage on Use of Service by Medicare Enrollees," *Health Care Financing Review* 19, no. 1 (Fall 1997), 5–18, U.S. Department of Health and Human Services.

9. Frank Lichtenberg, "Pharmaceutical Innovation, Mortality Reduction and Economic Growth," National Bureau of Economic Research, NBER Working Paper W6569, May 1998.

10. James D. Lubitz, and Gerald F. Riley, "Trends in Medicare Payments in the Last Year of Life," *New England Journal of Medicine* 328, no. 15 (April 15, 1993): 1092–96.

11. Andrew J. Rettenmaier and Thomas R. Saving, "Reforming Medicare," National Center for Policy Analysis, Policy Report No. 261, May 2003.

12. Rettenmaier and Saving, "Reforming Medicare."

13. Woolhandler, Campbell and Himmelstein, "Costs of Health Care Administration in the United States and Canada."

14. Patricia M. Danzon, "Hidden Overhead Costs: Is Canada's System Really Less Expensive?" *Health Affairs* 11, no. 1 (Spring 1992), 21–43.

15. Mark Litow and the Technical Committee of the Council for Affordable Health Insurance, "Rhetoric vs. Reality: Comparing Public and Private Health Care Administrative Costs," Council for Affordable Health Insurance, March 1994.

16. See John C. Goodman, "Characteristics of an Ideal Health Care System," National Center for Policy Analysis, Policy Report No. 242, April 2001.

17. Matt Hamblen, "Smart Cards Enter Health Care Community," *Enterprise Network News*, December 9, 1997. For a white paper on smart card technology, see Soon-Yong Choi and Andrew B. Whinston, "Smart Cards: Enabling Smart Commerce in the Digital Age," KPMG and the Center for Research in Electronic Commerce, University of Texas at Austin, May 1998, available at http://cism.bus.utexas.edu/works/articles/smartcardswp.html.

18. Thomas A. Massaro and Yu-Ning Wong, "Medical Savings Accounts: The Singapore Experience," National Center for Policy Analysis, Policy Report No. 203, April 1996. Also see Mukul G. Asher, "Compulsory Savings in Singapore: An Alternative to the Welfare State," National Center for Policy Analysis, Policy Report No. 198, September 1995.

19. Shaun Matisonn, "Medical Savings Accounts in South Africa," National Center For Policy Analysis, Policy Report no. 234, June 2000.

20. Cheryl Jackson, "Insurers Test Direct-Deposit Pay For Claims" *American Medical News* 44, no. 12 (March 26, 2001.

21. Tom Spring, "Put Your Medical Records Online. Doctors Launch a Private Medical Registry to Provide Patient Information in Emergencies," *PC World* (December 3, 1998). Also see Elisa Batista, "The Push for Online Medical Info," *Wired News* (May 9, 2000).

22. Joseph Conn, "Instant Response: Online Claims Authorization System Speeds Up Resolution," *Modern Physician* 4, no. 12 (December 1, 2000), 12–13.

23. See John C. Goodman and Gerald L. Musgrave, "Controlling Health Care Costs with Medical Savings Accounts," NCPA Policy Report No. 168, National Center for Policy Analysis, January 1992.

24. Ron Lieber, "Employers Offer New Pretax Perk," *Wall Street Journal*, September 2, 2003. For awhile there was a question about whether the IRS would allow medical expenses paid with a debit card to be tax-exempt without prior approval by a plan administrator. The IRS settled this question with a favorable revenue ruling.

25. Victoria Craig Bunce, "Medical Savings Accounts: Progress and Problems under HIPAA," Cato Institute, Policy Analysis No. 11, August 8, 2001.

26. Jon R. Gabel, Anthony T. Lo Sasso, and Thomas Rice, "Consumer-Driven Health Plans: Are They More Than Talk Now?" *Health Affairs* (November 20, 2002) (Web exclusive).

27. The deductibles are $1,000 per individual, $2,000 per family.

28. For a discussion of HRAs, see Devon Herrick, "Health Reimbursement Arrangements: Making a Good Deal Better," NCPA Brief Analysis No. 438, National Center for Policy Analysis, May 8, 2003.

Chapter Eleven

Priorities

MYTH NO. 11: UNDER SINGLE-PAYER NATIONAL HEALTH INSURANCE, HEALTH CARE DOLLARS WOULD BE ALLOCATED SO THAT THEY HAD THE GREATEST IMPACT ON HEALTH

The one characteristic of foreign health care systems that strikes American observers as the most bizarre is the way in which limited resources are allocated. Foreign governments do not merely deny lifesaving medical technology to patients under national insurance schemes. They also take money that could be spent saving lives and curing disease and spend it serving people who are not seriously ill. Often, the spending has little if anything to do with health care.

For example, the German health system spends billions of dollars on what amounts to paid holidays. Up to nine million Germans annually take month-long respites at spas and health resorts paid for by insurers. Some Germans were outraged in 2003 when the health minister announced plans to cut this benefit—as well as free cooking classes and taxi rides.[1] While billions of health care dollars are diverted for these frivolities, hospital care and drug therapies are rationed.[2]

SPENDING PRIORITIES IN BRITAIN

The tendency throughout the British NHS is to divert funds from expensive care for the small number who are seriously ill toward the large number who seek relatively inexpensive services for minor ills. Take British ambulance service, for example. British "patients" take between eighteen and nineteen million ambulance rides each year—about one ride for every three people in Britain.[3] Almost 80 percent of these rides are for such nonemergency purposes as taking an outpatient to a hospital or a senior to a pharmacy and amount to little more than free taxi service.

While thousands of people die each year from lack of kidney dialysis, the NHS provides an array of comforts for chronically ill people with less serious health problems. As tables 11.1 and 11.2 shows, the NHS provides nonmedical services to about 1.5 million people a year. These include day care services to more than 260,000, home care or home help services to 578,000, home alterations for 375,000 and occupational therapy for 456,000.[4]

In our study of the British NHS a decade ago, we wrote[5]

If the NHS did nothing more than charge patients the full costs of their sleeping pills and tranquilizers, enough money would be freed to treat 10,000 to 15,000 additional cancer patients each year and save the lives of an additional 3,000 kidney patients. Yet such options are not seriously considered.

Although we have not updated those calculations, it would appear that there has been little change in NHS priorities in the interim.

More than one million people are waiting to be admitted to NHS hospitals,[6] but the equivalent of 1,692 full-time doctors are tied up waiting for patients

TABLE 11-1

Nonmedical Spending by the British National Health Service

	Per Year
Nonemergency ambulance rides*	15,000,000
Missed physician appointments**	10,000,000
Patients receiving nonmedical services***	1,500,000

* Only 4 million rides were classified as emergency or urgent.

** The estimated cost of missed GP appointments is $250 million dollars.

*** Community services include meals on wheels, home care, day care, home adaptations and professional support.

Source: "Community Care Statistics 2000/2001, Referrals, Assessments and Packages of Care for Adults," UK Department of Health, 2001, Table P2f.1

TABLE 11-2

Nonmedical Services by the
British National Health Services
(Number of community services performed)

Home alterations	375,000
Occupational therapy	456,000
Day care services	260,000
Home care/home help services	578,000

Source: "Community Care Statistics 2000/2001, Referrals, Assessments and Packages
of Care for Adults," UK Department of Health, 2001, Table P2f.1.

who do not appear for appointments or call to cancel.[7] If the NHS did nothing more than charge patients the full costs of missed appointments, it would free up enough money to treat thousands of additional cancer patients each year. Yet, again, such options are not seriously considered.[8]

SPENDING PRIORITIES: GENERAL
PRACTITIONERS VERSUS SPECIALISTS

Another indicator of spending priorities is the degree to which countries allow physicians to specialize. In general, countries with national health insurance tend to encourage routine medical services for the vast majority of people who are healthy at the expense of specialized care for the few who are seriously ill. While only 11 percent of American physicians are engaged in general practice or family practice,[9]

- In Canada, just over half of all physicians are GPs.[10]
- In New Zealand, nearly half of all physicians are GPs.[11]
- Approximately two in three Australian physicians are GPs.[12]

In general, Canadians have little trouble seeing a GP. But specialist services and sophisticated equipment are increasingly rationed. In 2003, for example, Canadians waited an average of 8.3 weeks to see a specialist. However, as noted above, waiting can be much longer depending upon the province and the type of specialist. For instance, the median wait to see an orthopedic surgeon is 13.3 weeks for an initial consultation, with an additional wait of 18.9 weeks for treatment. This makes for a total wait of almost eight months.[13]

NOTES

1. Jane Burgermeister, "Germany Reaches Controversial Deal on Health Care Reform," *British Medical Journal* 327, no. 7409 (August 2, 2003), 250; and "Cuts Planned for German Spa Treatments," *British Medical Journal* (July 13, 1996) 313, no. 7049/72.

2. Annette Tuffs, "Germany at Center of Rationing Row as Budget in Crisis," *British Medical Journal* 313, No. 7049/72 (August 23, 2003) 317, no. 7412/414.

3. "Statistical Bulletin—Ambulance Services, England: 2000–2001," UK Department of Health, 2001, Table 1.

4. "Community Care Statistics 2000–2001, Referrals, Assessments and Packages of Care for Adults," UK Department of Health, 2001, Table P2f.1. Although most of these services are for the elderly, some adults between the ages of 18 and 64 are clients as well. For instance, home alterations are procedures designed to assist both the elderly and the disabled living at home, as are home care services. Occupational therapy is related to teaching and maintaining life skills, while day care and home care services allow the elderly or disabled to be cared for at home. See www.doh.gov.uk/public/comcare2001/tablep2f1.pdf.

5. Goodman and Musgrave, "Twenty Myths about National Health Insurance."

6. "Waiting List Figures, November 2001," UK Department of Health.

7. Patients miss an estimated 10 million general practitioner appointments totaling more than 2.5 million hours each year. Survey published by the Doctor Patient Partnership and Institute of Healthcare Management, August 14, 2001.

8. Some physicians have called for a flat £10 charge—approximately $14 to $15—to provide patients with an incentive to keep appointments, but the British Medical Association is opposed.

9. *Occupational Outlook Handbook*, Bureau of Labor Statistics, U.S. Department of Labor, 2002–2003 Edition, Physicians and Surgeons, Percent Distribution of M.D.s by Specialty, 1999, Table 1, January 2002.

10. National Information, Southam Medical Database, Canadian Institute for Health Information, 2002.

11. *New Zealand Workforce Statistics, 2000*, Medical Practitioners, New Zealand Health Information Service, 2000.

12. "Australian Social Trends, Health—Health Services: Distribution of General Practitioners," Australian Bureau of Statistics, 1994. This is the most recent available count by the Australian Bureau of Statistics.

13. Nadeem Esmail and Michael Walker, "Waiting Your Turn: Hospital Waiting Lists in Canada, 13th Edition," *Fraser Institute, Critical Issues Bulletin,* October 2003.

Chapter Twelve

Prevention

A common argument for national health insurance is that when care is "free" at the point of service people will more readily seek preventive services. Consequently, it is argued, money will be saved when doctors catch conditions in their early stages, before they develop into more costly-to-treat diseases. Yet, it turns out that patients in government-run health care systems do not get more preventive care than Americans do. And even if they did, that would not save the government money.

PREVENTION VERSUS PREVENTIVE CARE

A distinction should be made between "prevention" and "preventive medical care." Anything that can prevent a disease can be labeled prevention. This can include eating a proper diet, getting adequate exercise, losing excess weight, abstaining from smoking, drinking only in moderation and proper personal sanitation. Preventive medical care, on the other hand, is a much narrower concept. It includes regular exams and screening tests designed to catch a disease or a health problem in its early stages. It also covers medical interventions, such as vaccinations, designed to protect against disease. Most of the time, preventive care is like a *consumer good* that creates benefits in return for a cost; it is not like an *investment good* that promises a positive economic rate of return.

119

Poor lifestyle choices are responsible for a significant portion of the burden of disease on society. Better choices reduce the incidence of disease and disability. National health expenditures would be lower if everyone practiced prevention through adopting healthy lifestyles. For example, we now know that prevention of heart disease and strokes through lifestyle changes is possible. The same appears to be true of much diabetes and many cancers.

Most of the greatest public health triumphs in the twentieth century relate to prevention. In fact, according to public health experts, most of the increases in life expectancy over the last 100 years have resulted from improvements in public health rather than advances in medicine. These include such public health efforts as providing clean drinking water and improving sanitation. Worldwide, only a few medical advances, such as vaccination, have contributed to an overall increase in longevity.[1]

DO PREVENTIVE SERVICES SAVE MONEY?

Careful studies show that preventive medicine generally raises rather than lowers overall health care costs. As one observer put it, "nearly every aspect of preventive care has crashed upon the rocky shore of added costs."[2] Vaccination is one of the few preventive medical interventions that saves more money than it costs.[3] Very few medical procedures, including preventive or diagnostic procedures, pay for themselves in terms of a net lifetime reduction in total health care costs.[4] A study by the U.S. Office of Technology Assessment found only three kinds of preventive care save money: prenatal care for poor women, tests in newborns for certain congenital disorders and most childhood immunizations.[5] Other studies indicate that smoking cessation advice is another.[6]

However, Pap smears do not save money. Nor do mammograms. Nor do most other tests.[7] It is true that diagnosing cancer early lowers treatment costs for the patient found to have the disease. But in order to find that patient through screening, the diagnostic test must be given to thousands of healthy patients. When all costs are considered, the extra costs of screening the healthy swamp the reduced costs of treating the few found to have the disease.[8]

That preventive care usually adds to overall health care costs does not mean that it is not valuable. For instance, diagnostic tests showing that no disease is present benefits patients by relieving anxiety and creating the reassurance of health. But we need to compare the money spent with the benefits received. Take breast cancer, for example. Figure 12.1 shows the cost of screening, including the costs of treatment for those discovered to have cancer, per year of

FIGURE 12-1

Yearly Mammograms:
Cost per Year of Life Saved

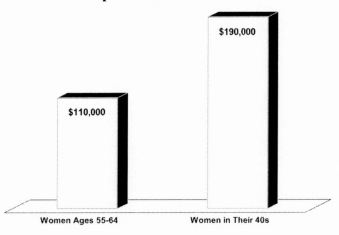

Source: Tammy O. Tengs et al., "Five Hundred Lifesaving Interventions and Their Cost-Effectiveness," *Risk Analysis*, June 1995.

life saved as a result of the screening and subsequent treatment for breast cancer. As the figure shows, giving regular mammograms to women age fifty-five to sixty-four costs about $110,000 for every year of life saved as a result of the screening, when all costs are considered. For women in their forties, the costs jump considerably, to $190,000 for each year of life saved.

This does not mean that mammograms are wasteful. To the contrary, they are a reasonable investment for many women. Economists have found that the price people are willing to pay to avoid various risks is in the range of $75,000 to $150,000 for each year of life saved.[9] Note that this is not the amount of money people are willing to pay to purchase an extra year of life. These numbers are *implied* by the amounts people are willing to pay to avoid risk when the risk is small and the amount of money also is small, such as the extra wages required to induce people to work in riskier jobs. Since the trade-offs for mammograms shown in the figure are near or in this range, regular mammograms are probably worthwhile for most women.

Similar considerations apply to some Pap smear exams for cervical cancer. Figure 12.2 shows the following:

• Screening young women every four years for cervical cancer costs less than $12,000 for each year of life saved.

FIGURE 12-2

Cervical Cancer Tests:
Cost per Year of Life Saved
(Women age 20)

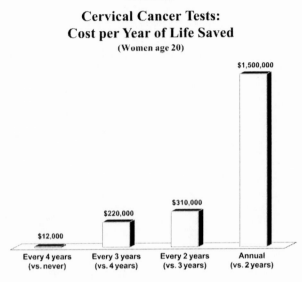

Source: Tammy O. Tengs et al., "Five Hundred Lifesaving Interventions and Their Cost-Effectiveness." *Risk Analysis*, June 1995.

- More frequent screening causes the costs to soar from about $220,000 per year of life saved at three-year intervals (as opposed to four-year intervals) to about $310,000 at two-year intervals (as opposed to three).
- Giving Pap smears every year (as opposed to every other year) is really expensive: almost $1.5 million per year of life saved.

Pap smear screening, even every fourth year, costs money; it does not save money. However, four-year cervical cancer tests are a very good buy in the business of risk avoidance. To put this figure in perspective, we note that there is a better payoff from wearing seatbelts in automobiles. But four-year cervical cancer testing is a better buy than air bags. More frequent screenings, however, make the costs rise rapidly in relation to the benefits. Despite the preference of many doctors for annual screening, the trade-off is well outside the range of choices people make to avoid risk in other walks of life.

Now suppose we ignore costs and ask: What is the right number of Pap smears from a purely medical point of view? There is no right answer. Four-year Pap smears produce a medical benefit. Annual Pap smears produce a bigger benefit. One presumes that monthly Pap smears would further enhance the benefit. Medical science alone cannot justify one frequency over any other, unless one adopts the untenable position that people should obtain any and all diagnostic tests that offer any possible medical benefit.

PREVENTIVE CARE IN THE UNITED KINGDOM

One might suppose that a system of "free" public health care would offer more preventive medicine. After all, if people face no financial deterrent to doctor visits, they should be more likely to take advantage of diagnostic tests that can detect diseases in their early states. Yet, there is no evidence that this happens. For example, estimates are that one out of every two diabetics goes undiagnosed[10] both in the United States and in Britain.

Preventive care may, in fact, be less available under a single-payer system because care *is* free. A comparison of American and British physicians in the 1990s found that the British saw a physician almost as often as Americans (about six times a year).[11] Yet, when Americans did see a doctor, the consultation was six times as likely to last more than twenty minutes (see figure 12.3).[12] A recent survey of 200 British GPs and more than 2,000 consumers found that 87 percent of smokers want more advice and help in quitting from their GPs. But 93 percent of GPs say they lack the time to give such advice.[13] A similar problem apparently exists in all countries. An *American Journal of Public Health* study concluded that if general internists with an average panel of adult patients provided all the recommended preventive care, that care would consume most of their days.[14]

Because Britons perceive doctor visits to be free, an inordinate proportion of their physician visits are for trivial complaints. To handle the caseload, British doctors spend less time with each patient. Moreover, as discussed above, British physicians have much less access to diagnostic equipment and must send their patients to hospitals even for chest X-rays and simple blood tests. Britain did not offer breast cancer screening until the late 1980s to early 1990s. The high breast cancer mortality rate in Britain may to some extent reflect the lack of screenings in the past.[15]

PREVENTIVE CARE IN CANADA

Physician time constraints are also a problem in Canada. On a per capita basis, Canadians visit physicians 10 percent more often than Americans do, but it is not clear that they receive more services. Apparently, more Canadian physician time is spent on (arguably) trivial conditions such as colds, sore throats or upset stomachs.[16] As figure 12.3 suggests, patients spend more time with physicians in the United States than in Canada.[17] Also, in Canada, fee structures are designed to discourage physicians from providing office-based procedures. The only office-based work physicians can bill for is the time they spend examining and evaluating patients. They cannot bill for diagnostic tests.[18]

FIGURE 12-3

Patients Spending More than
20 Minutes with Their Doctor

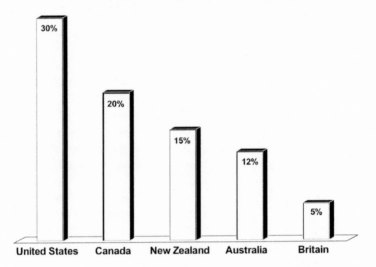

Note: Reflects most recent doctor visit.

Source: Karen Donelan et al., "The Cost of Health System Change: Public Discontent in Five Nations," *Health Affairs*, May/June 1999.

The amount of preventive care people get under single-payer systems appears to be based more on socioeconomic status and education than on whether medical care is free or not. For example, studies comparing women in Ontario and in two areas of the United States found that in both countries their chances of receiving a Pap smear or clinical breast cancer screening increased with education and income regardless of whether a woman had health insurance.[19]

INTERNATIONAL COMPARISON
OF CANCER PREVENTION

International comparisons are difficult at best, but there is evidence that problems exist in many countries with socialized health care systems. One international measure is "potential years of life lost" (PYLL) per 100,000 population.[20] This measure attempts to calculate the years of life lost needlessly because of a lack of preventive care. At 211 years of life lost for every

TABLE 12-1

Potential Life Years Lost To Breast Cancer
(per 100,000 people)

Canada	211
United States	214
France	224
Australia	226
Germany	232
United Kingdom	263
Netherlands	288
New Zealand	291
Ireland	291
Denmark	305

Note: Data is for 1997

Source: *OECD Health Data 2002.*

100,000 people, Canada edges out the U.S. rate of 214. At 224, 226 and 232, respectively, France, Australia and Germany are trailing. And many countries fare far worse, including 263 "life years" lost in Britain, 288 in the Netherlands, 291 in New Zealand and Ireland, and 305 in Denmark. As noted in chapter 6, a far higher proportion of women with breast cancer succumb to the disease in other countries than in the United States. The reasons for this are many, but poor screening programs may contribute.

NOTES

1. "10 Public Health Triumphs," *Nursing Library* (March 2000): 1; "Ten Great Public Health Achievements—United States, 1900–1999," *Morbidity and Mortality Weekly Report* 48, no. 12 (April 02, 1999): 241–43. For an in-depth review of each achievement, see the CDC's Web site at www.cdc.gov/od/oc/media/tengpha.htm.
2. Scott Gottlieb, "For HMOs, Preventive Medicine Doesn't Pay," *American Medical News* 44, no. 30 (August 13, 2001).
3. For a discussion of lifestyle changes that increase health and life expectancy, see N. B. Belloc and L. Breslow, "Relationship of Physical Health Status and Health Practice," *Preventive Medicine* 1 (1972): 409–21; Jack A. Meyer and Marion E. Lewin, "Introduction." In *Charting the Future of Health Care*, Meyer and Lewin, eds., (Washington, D.C.: American Enterprise Institute, 1987), 5; Bruce Bower, "Health Aging May

Depend on Past Habits," *Science News* 159, no. 24 (June 16, 2001); G.E. Vaillant and K. Mukamal, "Successful Aging," *American Journal of Psychiatry* 158 (June 2001), 839; Patricia Andersen-Parrado, "6 Strategies to Help You Live Longer and Better," *Better Nutrition* (April 2000); Hirofumi Shigeta, "Lifestyle, Obesity, and Insulin Resistance," *Diabetes Care* (March 2001); and Andrew Baum, "Health Psychology: Mapping Biobehavioral Contributions to Health and Illness," *Annual Review of Psychology* 50 (1999) 137–63.

4. Ashley B. Coffield et al., "Priorities among Recommended Clinical Preventive Services," *American Journal of Preventive Medicine* 21, no. 1 (2001) 66–67. For a comprehensive list of lifesaving interventions and their costs, see Tammy O. Tengs, "Dying Too Soon: How Cost-Effectiveness Analysis Can Save Lives," National Center for Policy Analysis, Policy Report No. 204, May 1997; and Tammy O. Tengs et al., "Five Hundred Lifesaving Interventions and Their Cost-Effectiveness," *Risk Analysis* 15, no. 3 (June 1995): 369–90.

5. U.S. Congress, Office of Technology Assessment, *Benefit Design in Health Care Reform: Report #1-Clinical Preventive Services* (Washington, D.C.: U.S. Government Printing Office, September 1993).

6. Tengs et al., "Five Hundred Lifesaving Interventions."

7. See "Is Preventive Medical Care Cost-Effective?" National Center for Policy Analysis, Brief Analysis No. 188, November 9, 1995. The Office of Technology Assessment (OTA) studied the cost-effectiveness of adding coverage for several preventive measures—including flu and pneumonia vaccines and screening tests for cervical and colon cancer—to the federal Medicare insurance program for the elderly. None of the preventive measures was found to cut costs. See U.S. Congress, Office of Technology Assessment, *Preventive Health Services for Medicare Beneficiaries: Policy and Research Issues* (Washington, D.C.: U.S. Government Printing Office, February 1990); and U.S. Congress, Office of Technology Assessment, *The Cost and Effectiveness of Colorectal Screening in the Elderly* (Washington, D.C.: U.S. Government Printing Office, September 1990).

8. See also "Is Preventive Medical Care Cost-Effective?" NCPA; and Louise B. Russell, *Is Prevention Better Than Cure?* (Washington, D.C.: Brookings Institution, 1986).

9. W. Kip Viscusi, "The Value of Risks to Life and Health," *Journal of Economic Literature* 31, no. 4 (December 1993): 1912–46; and George Tolley, Donald Kendel and Robert Fabian, eds., *Valuing Health for Policy: An Economic Approach* (Chicago: University of Chicago Press, 1994).

10. "Diabetes: Disabling, Deadly, and on the Rise, at a Glance 2002," National Center for Chronic Disease Prevention and Health Promotion, Centers for Disease Control, 2002, available at www.cdc.gov/diabetes/pubs/glance.htm. Also see Robin Turner, "Diabetes Test Aims to Trace Army of People Unaware that They are Sufferers," *Western Mail* (June 10, 2002); and "Who Get Diabetes and What Causes it?" *Diabetes U.K. 2000*, available at www.diabetes.org.uk/diabetes/get.htm.

11. Gerald F. Anderson and Jean-Pierre Poullier, "Health Spending, Access, and Outcomes: Trends In Industrialized Countries," *Health Affairs* 18, no. 3 (1999), 178–92.

12. See Edward W. Campion, "A Symptom of Discontent," *New England Journal of Medicine* 344, no. 3 (January 18, 2001): 223–25; and John G. R. Howie et al., "Quality at General Practice Consultations: Cross Sectional Survey," *British Medical Journal* 319, no. 7212 (September 18, 1999): 738–43. Note that the average general practitioner (GP) consultation was eight minutes in Britain, whereas the average consultation across all specialties in the United States was 18.3 minutes. See also David Mechanic, Donna D. McAlpine and Marsha Rosenthal, "Are Patients' Office Visits with Physicians Getting Shorter?" *New England Journal of Medicine* 344, no. 3 (January 18, 2001): 198–204.

13. "Challenging Nicotine Addiction," Smoking Cessation in Primary Care (SCRAPE), August 2001, reported in "U.K. Physicians Lack Time to Help Patients Quit Smoking," *Reuters Health*, August 23, 2001.

14. See Sandeep J. Jauhar, "That Ounce of Prevention Grew Too Big," *New York Times*, December 2, 2003; and Kimberly S. H. Yarnall et al., "Primary Care: Is There Enough Time for Prevention?," *American Journal of Public Health* 93, no. 4 (April 2003): 635–41.

15. J. Patnick, "Breast and Cervical Screening for Women in the United Kingdom," *Hong Kong Medical Journal* 6 (2000): 409–11.

16. Larry M. Greenberg, "Take Two Tablespoons of Mustard and Call If You Don't Feel Better," *Wall Street Journal*, February 22, 1994, cited in Rexford E. Santerre and Stephen P. Neun, *Health Economics: Theories, Insights, and Industry Studies* (Chicago: Irwin, 1996), 60.

17. Victor R. Fuchs and James S. Hahn, "How Does Canada Do It? A Comparison of Expenditures for Physicians' Service in the United States and Canada," *New England Journal of Medicine* 323, no. 13 (September 27, 1990): 884–90.

18. Patricia M. Danzon, "Hidden Overhead Costs: Is Canada's System Really Less Expensive?" *Health Affairs* 11, no. 1 (Spring 1992): 27.

19. See S. J. Katz and T. P. Hofer, "Socioeconomic Disparities in Preventive Care Persist Despite Universal Coverage: Breast and Cervical Cancer Screening in Ontario and the United States," *Journal of the American Medical Association* 272 (August 17, 1994): 530–34.

20. Potential years of life lost is a calculation that attempts to quantify preventable deaths and is weighted by age at death, with 70 being the maximum. If a person dies of a preventable death at 60, the potential numbers of life years lost would be 10. From *OECD Health Data 2002*.

Chapter Thirteen

Managed Care

**MYTH NO. 13: SINGLE-PAYER
NATIONAL HEALTH INSURANCE IS THE
SOLUTION TO THE PROBLEMS OF MANAGED CARE**

Although the term *managed care* means different things to different people, in all its guises it involves interference in the doctor-patient relationship by third-party bureaucracies (employers and insurance companies, for example) whose primary interest is in controlling costs. Most doctors and many patients want a different system. But would they really be better off under single-payer national health insurance? Because of doctors' frustrations with managed care, a national health system might seem appealing. Some believe it would reduce administrative paperwork, overhead costs and allow physicians to spend more time treating patients. However, physicians in countries with national health insurance also express frustration. They are able to spend even less time than U.S. physicians with each patient, face more obstacles to providing care and receive even less compensation. Despite American physicians' frustration with uninsured patients and managed care, these problems seem to pale in comparison with the lack of resources and bureaucratic hassles experienced by their national health insurance counterparts.

THE MANAGED CARE
REVOLUTION IN THE UNITED STATES

In 1980 fewer than ten million people were enrolled in HMOs. Today nearly seventy-two million are, about one in four Americans.[1] Three-fourths of all employees with health insurance are covered by some type of managed care. What difference has this change made?

For starters, it has meant fewer choices for patients and doctors. Only a few years ago, a person with private health insurance could see any doctor, enter any hospital or (with a prescription) obtain any drug. Today things are different. In general, patients must choose from a list of approved doctors covered by their health plans. Yet, employers switch health plans and, even if they don't, employees often switch jobs. So long-term relationships between patients and physicians are hard to form. Moreover, many people cannot see a specialist without a referral from a "gatekeeper" family physician or even get treatment at a hospital emergency room without prior (telephone) approval from their managed care organization. Patients who fail to follow the rules may have to pay part or all of the bill out of their own pockets.

Under managed care, freedom of choice has been curtailed even more for doctors than for patients. Not long ago, most doctors ordered tests, prescribed drugs, admitted patients to hospitals or referred them to specialists and performed procedures based on their own experience and professional judgment. No longer. Now doctors who want to be on the "approved" list must agree to practice medicine based on a health plan's guidelines. For most doctors, the guidelines mean fewer tests, fewer referrals and fewer hospital admissions. Since the advent of managed care, many doctors complain that they are under pressure to spend less time with each patient. Doctors also say they spend too much time and effort on billing, negotiating fees and interpreting insurance contracts.

How well has managed care succeeded in controlling costs? That's not clear. There is some evidence of success in the 1990s. But by the end of the decade, managed care plans faced a backlash from patients and doctors. In response, the plans began to loosen their control over patient access to specialists and expensive treatments and the rate of increase in health care costs began to rise.[2]

There is also evidence that people dislike the idea of managed care more than they dislike managed care itself. Polls show that, although 80 percent of people are satisfied with the care they receive from their HMO, 45 percent have negative opinions about HMOs in general.[3] Another recent survey tracked people who were unaware of their true insurance status. People who thought they were HMO members even if they were not were more likely to say they were dissatisfied than those who thought they were not in an HMO even though they were.[4]

EFFECTS OF SINGLE-PAYER
HEALTH INSURANCE ON PATIENTS

American advocates of single-payer health insurance say that such a system would resolve virtually all of the major abuses of managed care.[5]

Would it? Consider the principal patient criticisms of managed care: (1) you may not be able to see a specialist when you want to; (2) you might not be able to obtain expensive tests; (3) you may experience obstacles getting approval for surgery; and (4) you may have difficulty getting approval to enter a hospital. Yet, the problems American HMO enrollees face are minor compared to the hurdles faced by patients in other countries.

Almost all single-payer systems require patients to go through a gatekeeper who decides whether the patient gets a referral to a specialist. They also limit the number of specialists. Access to expensive technology is more difficult in single-payer systems than for patients in any managed care organization in the United States. Expensive technologies are rationed, including equipment necessary for diagnosis and treatment, such as MRIs. Admissions to hospitals are often cancelled or delayed.

As we noted in chapter 8, a recent study in the *British Medical Journal* compared services delivered by the British NHS with that of the California HMO, Kaiser Permanente. The study found the NHS provides far fewer services and less access to diagnostic tests and specialists than Kaiser, for only slightly less money.[6]

To make matters worse, advocates of single-payer insurance would take away an important right that all managed care patients currently have, the right to purchase their own care. Denied access to a specialist, U.S. patients can always go out of network and pay the cost themselves. Denied access to a diagnostic test, patients can pay for the test from their own resources. If the American advocates of single-payer insurance get their way, these private pay options will be outlawed.

EFFECTS OF SINGLE-PAYER HEALTH INSURANCE ON DOCTORS: LIMITING THE NUMBER OF PHYSICIANS

In countries with national health insurance, governments often attempt to limit demand for medical services by having fewer physicians.[7] Dr. Lorne Tyrrell, president of the Association of Canadian Medical Colleges, says Canada needs about 540 new physicians each year to account for population growth and another 1,950 to counter attrition.[8] However, since 1980 Canada has as a matter of policy reduced the number of students accepted by its sixteen medical schools to 1,577 per year, which is only 63 percent of the number it needs.[9]

There are approximately five qualified applicants for every one accepted to Canadian medical schools, and Canada has 25 percent fewer physicians per capita than the United States (see figure 13.1). Some students, unable to gain admission, have opted to study medicine in other countries. Despite the short-

FIGURE 13-1

Physicians per 1,000 People

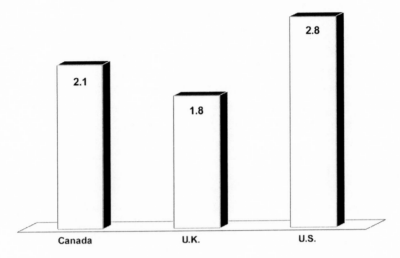

Source: Gerard F. Anderson, Uwe E. Reinhardt, Peter S. Hussey and Varduhi
Petrosyan, "It's the Prices, Stupid: Why the United States Is So
Different from Other Countries," *Health Affairs*, Vol. 22, No. 3, May/
June 2003, 89-105.

age of physicians, few of these foreign-trained Canadian doctors will ever be allowed to practice in Canada. Medical students are required to complete a Canadian residency program in order to practice there. But health authorities limit the number of residency slots to 100 for each 100 graduates of Canadian medical schools. For instance, the four medical schools in Quebec may only recruit a combined total of eight foreign medical graduates each year.[10] In most cases, the only way a foreign-trained physician can gain admission to a residency program is by promising to practice for a number of years in an underserved area.[11]

By contrast, about 16,000 students a year graduate from U.S. medical schools and enter graduate medical training. In addition, more than 5,100 foreign-trained medical graduates enter residency programs each year in the United States. Around 23 percent of these are U.S. citizens trained abroad while almost 40 percent are U.S. permanent residents. About one-third are non-U.S. citizens. There are virtually no restrictions on the number of graduate medical education programs, and no restrictions on the number of specialists.[12]

FIGURE 13-2

Patients Seen Annually

(Average per physician)

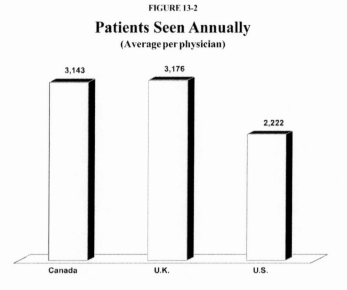

Source: Gerard F. Anderson and Peter S. Hussey, "Comparing Health System
Performance In OECD Countries," *Health Affairs*, May/June 2001.

EFFECTS OF SINGLE-PAYER HEALTH INSURANCE ON DOCTORS: MORE PATIENTS, LESS TIME

Because there are fewer physicians, doctors who practice medicine under single-payer systems must see larger numbers of patients for shorter periods of time. As figure 13.2 shows, U.S. physicians see an average of 2,222 patients per year, but physicians in Canada and Britain see an average of 3,143 and 3,176, respectively.[13] Family practitioners in Canada bear even higher patient loads—on the average, more than 6,000 per year.[14] Thus, it is not surprising that 30 percent of American patients spend more than twenty minutes with their doctor on a visit, compared to 20 percent in Canada and only 5 percent in Britain.[15]

In a recent survey, 30 percent of Canadians reported having difficulty finding a family physician. The survey also found that[16]

- Most family doctors' practices are full, and about 73 percent of all family practitioners do not routinely accept new patients.
- Of Canadian family physicians, more than 15 percent announced plans to stop practicing medicine in Canada in order to retire, practice in another country or for "other reasons" within the next two years.
- An additional 12.6 percent planned on taking a leave of absence or relocating their Canadian practice within the next two years.

The College of Family Physicians of Canada, which conducted the survey, concluded that the country needs 3,000 more family physicians now and predicted the shortage would worsen.

EFFECTS OF SINGLE-PAYER HEALTH INSURANCE ON DOCTORS: PHYSICIAN COMPENSATION

Like managed care organizations, one way single-payer systems try to reduce health expenditures is by squeezing the compensation of doctors, nurses and other health care workers. But a single-payer system can squeeze physicians' compensation much more effectively because it is a monopsony, a single buyer of a given good or service. Just as a monopoly seller can raise prices above the competitive market level, a monopsony buyer can reduce wages and fees below the market level.[17] As the Physicians' Working Group for Single-Payer National Health Insurance approvingly notes, "Such single source (monopsony) payment has been the cornerstone of cost containment and health planning in Canada and other nations with universal coverage."[18]

A Commonwealth Fund analysis compared physician incomes across countries after adjusting for differences in the cost of living. It found that doctors in other industrialized countries earn much less than those in the United States. As figure 13.3 shows, on the average doctors in Canada and Germany earn about

FIGURE 13-3

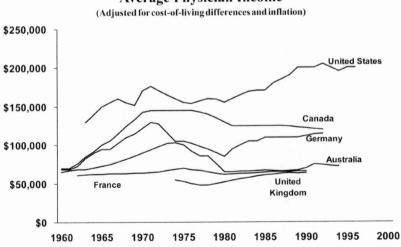

Average Physician Income
(Adjusted for cost-of-living differences and inflation)

Sources: Gerard F. Anderson, "Multinational Comparisons of Health Care: Expenditure, Coverage and Outcome," Commonwealth Fund, October 1998, and *OECD Health Data 1998*.

half as much; those in Australia, France and Britain earn less than one-third as much; and those in Finland, Norway, and Sweden earn one-fourth as much.[19]

Advocates also would discourage a physician's entrepreneurial activities. As proposed by Physicians for a National Health Insurance Program, for example, doctors would be paid a negotiated fee for their work and the services of their support staff. As a cost-saving measure to reduce "medical inflation," physicians would not be reimbursed for office-based procedures such as an MRI scan. The reason for this approach is to minimize "entrepreneurial incentives,"[20] a euphemism for profiting by meeting patient needs.

EFFECTS OF SINGLE-PAYER HEALTH INSURANCE ON DOCTORS: PHYSICIAN DISCONTENT IN BRITAIN

Dr. Michael Gross, a prominent neurologist, reported that he was on call 4,000 consecutive days at the Surrey & Sussex Healthcare Trust near London. After thirty-one years without a computer, and sharing one telephone with four other doctors, he finally resigned from the NHS when his neurological department was abolished.[21] His case is not surprising or isolated. Conditions in Britain's NHS are dismal by U.S. standards. British workloads are heavier and compensation is lower. Physicians have expressed growing dissatisfaction.[22] For example:

- In 2001, hundreds of family doctors announced plans to close their offices for a day to protest working conditions.[23]
- Between 20 percent and 25 percent of new doctors leave the NHS within five years of qualifying to practice medicine in Britain; many migrate to other countries or leave the medical profession altogether.[24]
- A study of medical graduates in Northwest England found that almost one-fifth had become disillusioned with the NHS and left over a ten-year period.[25]
- A survey of Scottish GPs found that 60 percent were considering leaving medicine for other careers because of working conditions.[26]

A BETTER ALTERNATIVE TO MANAGED CARE: HSAs[27]

As noted in the introduction, someone has to choose between health care and other uses of money. That someone may be: (1) a government-created bureaucracy, (2) a private-sector bureaucracy or (3) patients making their own decisions in consultation with doctors. The first is the method of single-payer national health insurance. The second is the method of managed care. And the third is envisioned in the creation of HSAs.

Even though savings accounts from which patients can pay medical bills directly have existed for a decade in South Africa[28] and for two decades in Singapore,[29] they are a relatively new idea in the United States. At the end of 2003, for example, only about 70,000 people had a tax-free MSA and an estimated 1.5 million had an HRA. The number of these accounts, which we described in chapter 10, is quite small for a country of almost 300 million people.

Despite our limited experience, the very idea of patient power generates intense opposition among people and organizations, ranging from Senator Edward Kennedy to Families USA to Consumers Union. We know from participation in public debates that critics often have very little direct knowledge about HSAs or similar accounts. They have never seen one. They have never owned one. They don't know anyone else who has ever owned one. But this lack of knowledge and experience has in no way tempered the knee-jerk zeal of the opponents.

Rhetoric aside, careful studies of the accounts do not bear out the arguments of the critics. Although critics claim people skimp on needed medical care in order to save money, the evidence shows otherwise. A Rand Health Insurance Experiment, conducted more than two decades ago, randomly assigned people to high-deductible (about $3,000 at today's prices) health plans and plans that made health care free of charge. Both groups had similar health outcomes even though those with high-deductible plans spent less on health care.[30] Similarly, a National Center for Policy Analysis study of South Africa found no evidence that MSA holders skimp on needed care.[31]

Although critics claim that HSAs will not control costs, in the Rand experiment patients with high deductibles spent about 30 percent less on health care. Similar results have been reported from South Africa.[32] For prescription drugs in particular, a second NCPA study concluded that patients managing their own health care funds saved just as much as those in managed care, but without the cost of managed care.[33]

Although critics claim that health accounts help only the healthy and the wealthy, studies also rebut this criticism. A separate Rand study found that when given a choice of MSAs or managed care plans, the families that chose MSAs had lower incomes and greater health care needs than families that chose managed care.[34] The Urban Institute has concluded, "on average, lower-wage workers would benefit from switching to MSA/catastrophic plans."[35] The NCPA's study of the South Africa experience concluded that MSA holders were not healthier as a group.[36]

Critics also charge that patients with health accounts will pay higher prices because they do not have the bargaining power of large institutional buyers.

Yet, in virtually all MSA plans, patients spending from their MSAs pay the same prices their third-party insurer pays — rates negotiated with provider networks. Even when they go outside of the network, patients spending their own money often pay lower prices than large insurers because doctors are willing to give discounts if they can avoid the costs of dealing with bureaucracies.

CASE STUDY: COSMETIC SURGERY

Prices for medical services have been rising faster than prices of other goods and services for as long as anyone can remember. But not all health care prices are rising. Although health care inflation is robust for those services paid by third-party insurance, prices are rising only moderately for services patients buy directly. As figure 13.4 shows, the real (inflation-adjusted) price of cosmetic surgery fell over the past decade, despite a huge increase in demand and considerable innovation.

FIGURE 13-4

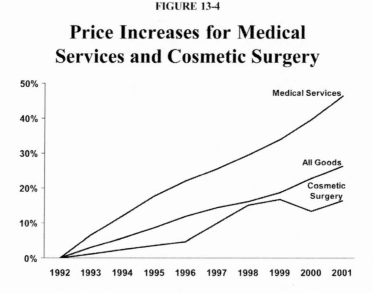

Price Increases for Medical Services and Cosmetic Surgery

Note: Cosmetic surgery index is calculated based on average price of common procedures weighted by their respective proportion of all cosmetic procedures. Procedures selected represent 54 percent of all cosmetic procedures performed.

Source: Authors' calculations using data from the Consumer Price Index (CPI) and the American Society of Plastic Surgeons.

Cosmetic surgery is one of the few types of medical care for which consumers pay almost exclusively out of pocket. Even so, the demand for cosmetic surgery exploded in recent years. Of the 6.6 million cosmetic procedures performed in 2002, 1.6 million were surgical procedures, nearly four times the number performed in 1992. Despite the quadrupling of the number of surgeries, cosmetic surgeons' fees remained relatively stable. What explains this price stability? One reason is patient behavior. When patients pay with their own money, they have an incentive to be savvy consumers. A second reason is supply. As more people demanded the procedures, more surgeons began to provide them. Since almost any licensed medical doctor may obtain training and perform cosmetic procedures, entry into the field is relatively easy. A third reason is efficiency. Many providers have operating facilities located in their offices, a less expensive alternative to outpatient surgery at a hospital. Surgeons generally adjust their fees to stay competitive and usually quote patients a package price. Absent are the gatekeepers, prior authorization and large medical office billing staffs needed when third-party insurance pays the fees. A fourth reason is the emergence of substitute products (see below).

Web sites help create a competitive market for cosmetic procedures. One, www.Bidforsurgery.com, is a reverse auction site that works much like eBay. Physicians submit competitive bids to perform procedures. The potential patient compares bids and quality indicators—information on residency, education, board certifications, and so forth. Patients can select a bid from among those physicians bidding or reject them all. If the patient does choose one of the bids, he or she gets a free consultation with the selected physician before making a final commitment.

A common perception is that innovation results in health care inflation. But in cosmetic surgery, innovation often lowers the cost. Take facelifts, for example. Surgical fees for facelifts increased only 20 percent between 1992 and 2001 (which in real terms is a price reduction), according to data from the American Society of Plastic Surgeons.

Holding the cost of facelift surgery in check were cheaper procedures designed to reduce the appearance of aging. Laser resurfacing ($2,232) can replace or delay surgical facelifts in some patients. Retin-A treatments ($124 per visit), botox injections ($388), collagen injections ($333), chemical peels ($516), dermabrasion ($1,254) and fat injection ($1,053) are other facelift alternatives. These less invasive (and less expensive) procedures may be attractive, compared to a facelift costing $5,007 in surgeons' fees alone. Cosmetic surgeons also have incentives to find new products to meet customer needs. Laser hair removal, for example, is now common.

The contrast between cosmetic surgery and other medical services is important. One sector has a competitive marketplace and stable prices. The other does not.

NOTES

1. *The InterStudy Competitive Edge: HMO Industry Report 13.2* (St. Paul, Minn: InterStudy, 2003). HMO enrollment figures as of January 1, 2003, and *Medicare Managed Care Market Penetration Report, All Medicare Plans*, Centers for Medicare and Medicaid Services, June 2000.

2. Alain Enthoven and Sara J. Singer, "The Managed Care Backlash and the Task Force in California," *Health Affairs* 17, no. 4 (July/August 1998): 95–110. Also see Robert J. Blendon et al., "Understanding the Managed Care Backlash," *Health Affairs* 17, no. 4 (July/August 1998): 80–94.

3. Gary Langer, "Conflicting Views on HMOs," *ABCNEWS.com,* January 22, 1999.

4. James D. Reschovsky and J. Lee Hargraves, "Health Care Perceptions and Experiences: It's Not Whether You Are In an HMO, It's Whether You Think You Are," Center for Studying Health System Change, Issue Brief #30, September 2000.

5. Don R. McCanne, "Would Single-Payer Health Insurance Be Good for America?" Physicians for a National Health Program, March 27, 2000.

6. Richard G. A. Feachem, Neelam K. Sekhri and Karen L. White, "Getting More for Their Dollar: A Comparison of the NHS with California's Kaiser Permanente," *British Medical Journal*, January 19, 2002, 143. Also see Alain Enthoven, "Commentary: Competition Made Them Do It," *British Medical Journal* 324, no. 7330 (January 19, 2002): 143.

7. This theory is sometimes referred to as "physician-induced demand" whereby an increase in the number of physicians is thought to increase demand for medical care since physicians are supposedly in a position to provide unknowledgeable patients with more care than is necessary.

8. Patrick Sullivan, "Concerns about Size of MD Workforce, Medicine's Future Dominate CMA Annual Meeting," *Canadian Medical Association Journal* 161, no. 5 (September 7, 1999): 561–62.

9. Greg L. Stoddart and Morris L. Barer, "Will Increasing Medical School Enrollment Solve Canada's Physician Supply Problems?" *Canadian Medical Association Journal* 161, no. 8 (October 19, 1999): 983–84. For an in-depth report of physician supply in Canada, see Lorne Tyrrell et al. (Canadian Medical Forum Task Force on Physician Supply in Canada), "Task Force on Physician Supply in Canada," November 22, 1999, available at www.cpsbc.ca/physician/publications/supply.pdf. Accessed December 2003.

10. Charlotte Gray, "How Bad Is the Brain Drain?" *Canadian Medical Association Journal* 161, no. 8 (October 19 1999): 1028–29.

11. Patrick Sullivan, "Shut Out at Home, Canadians Flocking to Ireland's Medical Schools—and to an Uncertain Future," *Canadian Medical Association Journal* 162, no. 6 (March 21, 2000): 868–71.

12. See Rebecca S. Miller, Marvin R. Dunn and Thomas Richter, "Graduate Medical Education, 1998–1999: A Closer Look," *Journal of the American Medical Association* 282, no. 9 (September 1, 1999): 855–60.

13. Gerard Anderson and Peter Sotir Hussey, "Comparing Health System Performance in OECD Countries," *Health Affairs* 20, no. 3 (May/June 2001): 219–32.

14. According to a survey, Canadian family physicians see an average of 124 patients per week. See Pat Rich, "Seventy Percent of Country's FP Practices Closed to New Patients: Survey," *Canadian Medical Association Journal* 65, no. 11 (November 27, 2001).

15. Karen Donelan et al., "The Cost of Health System Change: Public Discontent in Five Nations," *Health Affairs* 18, no. 3 (May/June 1999) 206–16.

16. Updated Data Release of the "2001 National Family Physician Workforce Survey," College of Family Physicians of Canada, August 2002.

17. Mark V. Pauly, "Managed Care, Market Power, and Monopsony," *Health Services Research* 33, no. 5 (December 1998): 1439–60.

18. Physicians' Working Group on Single-Payer National Health Insurance, "Proposal for Health Care Reform."

19. Anderson, "Multinational Comparisons of Health Care." Also see Gerard F. Anderson and Jean-Pierre Poullier, "Health Spending, Access, and Outcomes: Trends In Industrialized Countries," *Health Affairs* 8, no. 3 (1999).

20. Marcia Angell et al., Physicians' Working Group on Single-Payer National Health Insurance, "Proposal for Health Care Reform," Presentation to the Congressional Black Caucus and the Congressional Progressive Caucus, May 1, 2001.

21. Jeevan Vasagar, "NHS in Chaos from Top Down, Says Consultant," *Guardian Unlimited*, July 5, 2001, 5.

22. For more on physician morale, see M. McBride and D. Metcalfe, "General Practitioners' Low Morale: Reasons and Solutions," *British Journal of General Practice* 45 (1995): 227–29; R. Petchey, "Exploratory Study of General Practitioners' Orientations to General Practice and Responses to Change," *British Journal of General Practice* 44 (1994): 551–55; B. Leese and N. Bosanquet, "Changes in General Practice Organization: Survey of General Practitioners' Views on the 1990 Contract and Fundholding," *British Journal of General Practice* 46 (1996): 95–99.

23. "GPs Plan Day of Protest over Working Conditions," *Ananova.com*, May 1, 2001.

24. John Crace, "Health Scare: As a Medical Career Becomes Less Popular, Where Will New Doctors Come From?" *Guardian Unlimited*, December 4, 2001.

25. "Poor Working Conditions Force Doctors out of NHS," *BBC News*, June 10, 1998.

26. Gaby Hinsliff, "Young GPs Will Get Golden Hello," *Guardian Unlimited*, March 11, 2001.

27. See Michael Cannon, "Answering the Critics of Health Accounts," National Center Policy Analysis, Brief Analysis No. 454, September 12, 2003.

28. Shaun Matisonn, "Medical Savings Accounts in South Africa," National Center For Policy Analysis, Policy Report no. 234, June 2000.

29. Thomas A. Massaro and Yu-Ning Wong, "Medical Savings Accounts: The Singapore Experience," National Center for Policy Analysis, NCPA Policy Report No. 203, April 1996.

30. See Robert Brook et al., *The Effect of Coinsurance on the Health of Adults* (Santa Monica, Calif.: Rand, 1984); and Willard Manning et al., "Health Insurance and the Demand for Health Care: Evidence from a Randomized Experiment," *American Economic Review* 77, no. 3 (June 1987), 251–77. The Rand study was conducted from 1974 to 1982. A $1,000 deductible over that period would be equivalent to a deductible between $1,899 and $3,718 today. The one exception was vision care, which is not surprising since eyeglasses are often viewed as an elective health care expenditure.

31. Matisonn, "Medical Savings Accounts in South Africa."

32. Matisonn, "Medical Savings Accounts in South Africa."

33. Shaun Matisonn, "Medical Savings Accounts and Prescription Drugs: Evidence from South Africa," National Center for Policy Analysis, Policy Report No. 254, June 2000.

34. Dana P. Goldman, Joan L. Buchanan and Emmett B. Keeler, "Simulating the Impact of Medical Savings Accounts on Small Business," Rand Corporation, *HSR: Health Services Research* 35, no. 1, Part 1 (April 2000): 53–75.

35. Len M. Nichols et al., "Tax Preferred Medical Savings Accounts and Catastrophic Health Insurance Plans: A Numerical Analysis of Winners and Losers," Urban Institute, April 1996.

36. Matisonn, "Medical Savings Accounts in South Africa."

Chapter Fourteen

International Competitiveness

MYTH NO. 14: A SINGLE-PAYER NATIONAL HEALTH CARE SYSTEM WOULD IMPROVE U.S. COMPETITIVENESS IN INTERNATIONAL MARKETS AND BENEFIT AMERICAN WORKERS

Nearly two-thirds of Americans receive health care coverage through their employer. Some critics argue that the high health care costs borne by employers make U.S. products less competitive in the international marketplace and therefore harm American workers.[1] They assert that the cost of employer-provided health insurance adds to the price of American products, whereas a single-payer system would make American manufacturers more competitive by relieving employers of those costs. However, these assertions are wrong.

There is no evidence that the cost of private health insurance adds anything to the price of goods and services sold in the marketplace.[2] Health insurance is simply one element in a workers' total compensation package. It is a nontaxable fringe benefit provided to workers in lieu of money wages. Benefits for most American workers have grown from less than 19 percent of payroll in 1951 to nearly 39 percent today.[3] This reflects the fact that workers, faced with taxes on wage income, have increasingly preferred to receive a larger portion of their compensation in the form of nontaxed benefits.[4] However, workers' total compensation depends on what they produce, not what they consume.

The fact that Americans spend a greater proportion of their income on health care and a smaller proportion on other goods and services does not put us at a competitive disadvantage relative to other countries.[5] The same principle applies to other countries. For example, the Japanese spend a greater proportion of their income on food, but that doesn't mean that food consumption adds to the price of a Japanese car. Canadians spend a greater proportion of their income on education, but that doesn't mean that education adds to the price of Canadian lumber. These international differences merely reflect consumer preferences and consumer product prices.

A single-payer health insurance system, however, would reduce our international competitiveness. Consider the impact such systems have already had on the competitiveness of European countries. Taxes are a higher percentage of national income in all of these countries than in the United States, and health expenditures are a higher proportion of government budgets. High tax burdens are associated with lower rates of economic growth, job creation and income. Thus, national health insurance has contributed to high unemployment and increasing labor costs in Europe.

Health insurance benefits voluntarily provided by employers do not raise their labor costs. But when employers are required to pay the government for each worker they employ at a rate that bears no relation to the cost of health care consumed by those employees or the value of their work, it raises an employer's labor costs. For example, Germany's sickness insurance funds are financed by compulsory contributions of 13.5 percent of payroll, shared equally by employers and employees.[6] In France, health care is financed by a payroll tax of 12.8 percent on employers and 0.75 percent on employees; additionally, employees pay 7.5 percent of all income (including interest, dividends and other earnings) as a general social contribution, most of which goes to health insurance. Many also contribute an additional 2.5 percent to insurers for a total cost of more than 20 percent of payroll for health care.[7]

Not only would a single-payer health insurance system require additional taxes on American industries, it would also redistribute income among producers in different industries. On the whole, a single-payer health insurance system would impose extra taxes on U.S. exporting industries and use the proceeds of those taxes to subsidize other industries. The industries that would receive subsidies contribute mostly to domestic rather than international markets. The industries that would be penalized are the manufacturers that provide most of our exports.[8]

Almost a quarter of the federal budget goes to defense spending, whereas our trading partners spend far less. Yet, taxes are lower in the United States than in most other developed countries. As figure 14.1 shows, only Japan currently has a tax burden as low as ours.[9] Moreover, the United States regularly ranks as the most economically competitive nation in the world.[10] Evidently, the lack of single-payer health care has not harmed its ability to compete.

FIGURE 14-1

Tax Burden in the United States and Major Trading Partners[1]

(Tax revenue as a percent of GDP)

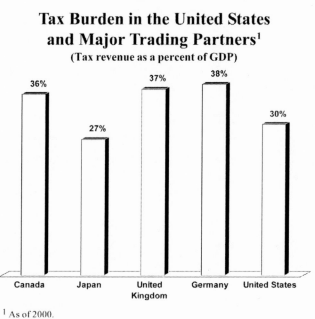

[1] As of 2000.

Source: Organization for Economic Cooperation and Development,
Revenue Statistics of OECD Member Countries, 2001 Edition,
July 2002.

NOTES

1. This argument is often based on the fact that most workers obtain their health insurance through their employer and Americans spend more on their health care system than other countries. For example, see Noam Chomsky, *Secrets, Lies and Democracy* (Tucson: Odonian Press, 1994).

2. Goodman and Musgrave, "Twenty Myths about National Health Insurance."

3. U.S. Chamber of Commerce, "Employee Benefits Historical Data 1951–1979" and Bureau of Labor Statistics, "Employer Costs for Employee Compensation—June 2003" News Release USDL: 03-446, Bureau of Labor Statistics, U.S. Department of Labor, August 26, 2003.

4. W. Michael Cox and Richard Alm, "The Economy's Good News: The Upside of Downsizing," National Center for Policy Analysis, *Policy Backgrounder,* no. 145, February 25, 1998.

5. For a discussion of health care spending and competitiveness, see Uwe Reinhardt, "Health Care Spending and American Competitiveness," *Health Affairs* 8, no. 4 (Winter 1989): 5–21.

6. Volker Ulrich, "Health Care in Germany: Structure, Expenditure and Prospects," Fraser Institute, October 10, 1999.

7. David G. Green in Robert E. Moffit et al., "Perspectives on the European Health Care Systems: Some Lessons for America," Heritage Foundation, Lecture No. 711, July 9, 2001. In Germany's two-tiered system, about 90 percent of the population pays the tax for insurance through sickness funds. But those whose income is above a certain level are allowed to opt out of the sickness funds and, instead of paying the tax, use the money to buy private insurance; about 10 percent have done so.

8. See the discussion in Goodman and Musgrave, "Twenty Myths about National Health Insurance."

9. *Revenue Statistics of OECD Member Countries, 2001 Edition* (Paris: OECD, 2002).

10. See "WCY Overall Scoreboard" and "Past Rankings," based on the *World Competitiveness Yearbook 2003* (Lausanne, Switzerland: IMD, 2003), available at http://www02.imd.ch/wcy/ranking.

Chapter Fifteen

The Elderly

MYTH NO. 15: SINGLE-PAYER NATIONAL HEALTH INSURANCE WOULD BENEFIT AMERICA'S ELDERLY

If the experience of other countries is any guide, the elderly have the most to lose under a national health insurance system. In general, when health care is rationed, the young get preferential treatment, while older patients get pushed to the rear of the waiting lines.

AGE DISCRIMINATION IN BRITAIN

Elderly Britons are generally able to schedule appointments with GPs and can usually gain access to medical facilities, albeit with difficulty. However, many do not receive the treatment and specialized care they need. Access to both emergency and nonemergency surgery is limited, as younger, healthier patients are given priority and allowed to pass seniors in the queue. In Britain, what is termed *ageism* has been discussed extensively in medical circles and in the popular media.[1]

- Extrapolating from a Gallup survey, the charity Age Concern estimated that one in ten people, or nearly two million, notice a difference in the way they are treated by the NHS after their fiftieth birthday.[2]
- One in twenty people over age sixty-five said they had been refused treatment; and many said their doctors told them the money would be better spent treating younger patients.[3]

- A British newspaper, *The Observer*, says, "[T]he NHS suffers from 'entrenched ageism,' with elderly patients receiving lower standards of care and less respectful treatment than the rest of the population."[4]
- Although more than one-third of all diagnosed cancers occur in patients seventy-five years of age or older, most cancer-screening programs in the NHS do not include people over age sixty-five.[5]
- The British Thoracic Society and the Society of Cardiothoracic Surgeons of Great Britain and Ireland reported that only one in fifty lung cancer patients over age seventy-five receives surgery.[6]
- In one particularly disturbing case, *BBC News* alleged that sixty seniors died after being deprived of food and water by hospital staff in an effort to free up hospital beds.[7]

Age discrimination is not just an action of individual doctors or hospital staff. In countries with single-payer health insurance systems, denial of care to the elderly is an institutional choice.[8] For example, guidelines issued by the British Medical Association allow NHS doctors to withdraw food and water given by tube to elderly patients suffering from severe stroke and dementia even if they are not facing imminent death.[9] In an effort to curb costs, the NHS has cut the number of geriatric beds in British hospitals by 50 percent over the past twenty years.[10]

Some NHS critics claim that its policies toward the elderly deliberately aim to eliminate the burden they place on the system and amount to a strategy of involuntary euthanasia.[11] This may help explain why the number of senior citizens deaths per capita from pneumonia is much higher in Britain than in the United States. For instance[12]:

- Deaths from pneumonia for patients between the ages of sixty-five and seventy-four are more than double in Britain compared to the United States.
- Almost three times as many British males aged seventy-five and above die of pneumonia than comparable American males—1,304 per 100,000 versus 492.
- More than three times as many British females aged seventy-five and above die of pneumonia than comparable American females—1,233 per 100,000 versus 385.

AGE DISCRIMINATION IN NEW ZEALAND

New Zealand's guidelines for end stage renal failure programs say that age should not be the sole factor in determining eligibility, but that "in usual cir-

FIGURE 15-1

How the Elderly Evaluate Their Health Care: Responses to Survey Questions

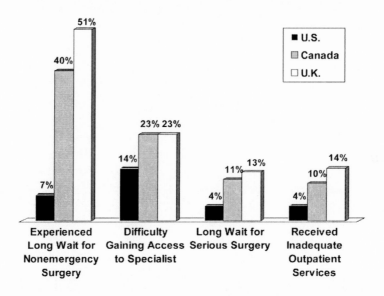

Source: Cathy Schoen et al., "The Elderly's Experiences with Health Care in Five
Nations," Commonwealth Fund, May 2000.

cumstances, people over seventy-five should not be accepted." Since New Zealand has no private dialysis facilities, this amounts to a death sentence for elderly patients with kidney failure.[13]

INTERNATIONAL COMPARISONS

How serious is the problem of restricted access to lifesaving care and medical technology for elderly patients? Lacking hard data, one can only speculate. As noted above, health economists are reluctant to take population mortality rates as an indicator of health care quality, at least among developed countries. Whether a person lives or dies in any given year is more likely a result of that person's lifestyle and environment than anything hospitals or doctors do.[14] Despite these caveats, if the health care system affects life expectancy in any population group, it is likely to be the elderly. International statistics on population mortality are consistent with the proposition that the elderly have the most to lose by nonprice rationing of medical care. According to one study,[15]

- Although there is very little relationship between health care spending and life expectancy at birth in OECD countries, at age eighty there is a significant correlation.
- An eighty-year-old U.S. female can expect to live almost a year longer than her British counterpart.
- An eighty-year-old U.S. male can expect to live a half-year longer than his British counterpart.

As the portion of the population that is elderly continues to grow in developed countries, seniors' access to health care in countries with a single-payer health insurance system is likely to deteriorate further. These countries will increasingly face the unpleasant choice of raising taxes or providing less care.

The vast majority of elderly citizens in the United States are enrolled in Medicare. As we note at several points in this book, this system is far from perfect. Nonetheless, with some exceptions discussed in chapter 1, Medicare gives seniors access to virtually all that the U.S. health care system has to offer. Compared to seniors in other countries, America's seniors experience fewer problems accessing care.[16] (See figure 15.1.)

Some have suggested creating a single-payer program in this country by letting everyone join Medicare. But that would be a disaster for the elderly. Under the current system, the federal government uses its monopsonistic bargaining power to pay what often amounts to below market prices for the services of doctors and hospitals.[17] Until now, however, providers have largely been able to cross subsidize—to make up for low Medicare payments by charging private payers more.[18] If everyone were in Medicare, no one would be left to shift costs to. Faced with too little reimbursement, providers would have to ration care. In that eventuality, elderly patients would almost certainly be pushed to the rear of the rationing lines.

NOTES

1. See, for example, J. Grimley Evans, "The Rationing Debate: Rationing Health Care by Age: The Case Against," *British Medical Journal* 314, no. 7083 (March 15, 1997): 822–25; Ann Bowling, "Ageism in Cardiology," *British Medical Journal* 319, no. 7221 (November 20, 1999): 1353–55; Graham C. Sutton, "Will You Still Need Me, Will You Still Screen Me, When I'm Past 64?" *British Medical Journal* (October 25, 1997): 1032–33; and Michael Rivlin, "Should Age-Based Rationing of Health Care Be Illegal?" *British Medical Journal* 319, no. 7221 (November 20, 1999), 1379.

2. Linda Beecham, "Patients Say the NHS Is Ageist," *British Medical Journal* (April 24, 1999): 1095; Celia Hall, "Campaign to Halt Ageism in NHS," *Daily Telegraph* (London), November 8, 1999.

3. Hall, "Campaign to Halt Ageism."

4. Kamal Ahmed, "Elderly Suffering 'Ageism' in NHS," *The Observer*, January 27, 2002. For the results of a survey on ageism in the NHS, see Caroline Gilchrist, "Too Old to Care," *The Guardian*, May 17, 2000.

5. Nicola J. Turner et al., "Cancer In Old Age: Is It Inadequately Investigated And Treated?," *British Medical Journal* 319, no. 7205 (July 31, 1999): 309–12. Also see Sutton, "Will You Still Need Me?"

6. Martyn R. Partridge, "Thoracic Surgery in a Crisis," *British Medical Journal* (February 16, 2001): 376–77.

7. "NHS Euthanasia Claims Ludicrous," *BBC News,* December 6, 1999.

8. Jammi N. Rao, "Politicians, Not Doctors, Must Make the Decisions about Rationing," *British Medical Journal* (April 3, 1999), 940.

9. "British Hospitals Deprive Elderly, Doctors Say," *BBC News,* December 6, 1999. Also see Sandra Laville and Celia Hall, "Elderly Patients 'Left Starving to Death in NHS,'" *Daily Telegraph* (London), December 6, 1999.

10. See report by the Counsel and Care Charity as reported in "Pensioners a Burden to NHS," *BBC News,* April 3, 1998.

11. "NHS Euthanasia Claims Ludicrous,'" *BBC News,* December 6, 1999.

12. Heinz Redwood, *Why Ration Care?* (London: CIVITAS, Institute for the Study of Civil Society, 2000).

13. Colin M. Feek et al., "Experience with Rationing Health Care in New Zealand," *British Medical Journal* 318, no. 7194 (May 15, 1999): 1346–48.

14. For a discussion of lifestyle and life expectancy, see Gary E. Fraser and David J. Shavlik, "Ten Years of Life: Is It a Matter of Choice?" *Archives of Internal Medicine* 161, no. 13 (July 9, 2001): 1645–52; Damaris Christensen, "Making Sense of Centenarians: Genes and Lifestyle Help People Live through a Century," *Science News* 159, no. 10 (March 10, 2001); Jack A. Meyer and Marion E. Lewin, "Introduction," *Charting the Future of Health Care* (Washington, D.C.: American Enterprise Institute, 1987), 5; Patricia Andersen-Parrado, "6 Strategies to Help You Live Longer and Better," *Better Nutrition* (April 2000); and Hirofumi Shigeta, "Lifestyle, Obesity, and Insulin Resistance," *Diabetes Care* (March 2001).

15. Anderson and Hussey, "Health and Population Aging: A Multinational Comparison."

16. Cathy Schoen et al., "The Elderly's Experiences with Health Care in Five Nations," Commonwealth Fund, May 2000.

17. Medicare physician fees were 83 percent of average private rates in 2001. See Kevin Hayes (Medicare Payment Advisory Commission) and Christopher Hogan (Direct Research, LLC), "Medicare Physician Payment Rates Compared to Rates Paid by the Average Private Insurer, 1999–2001," No. 0 3–6, Direct Research, LLC, August 27, 2003.

18. As the hospital marketplace has become more competitive, these cost shifting opportunities are diminishing.

Chapter Sixteen

Minorities

MYTH NO. 16: SINGLE-PAYER NATIONAL HEALTH INSURANCE WOULD BENEFIT RACIAL MINORITIES

Critics of the U.S. health care system often point to the disadvantages faced by minorities. On the average, African Americans and Hispanic Americans are less likely than whites to have health insurance, see a physician or enter a hospital. But is single-payer health insurance the answer? Empirical studies show that minorities also face medical discrimination under systems of national health insurance.[1] In fact, they often fare worse.

In a market where prices are used to allocate resources, goods and services are rationed by price. Willingness to pay, rather than race or political connections, determines which individuals utilize resources. In a nonmarket system, things are very different. Unable to discriminate on the basis of price, suppliers of services must discriminate among potential customers based on other factors. Race and ethnic background are invariably among those factors.[2]

RACIAL DISCRIMINATION IN THE UNITED STATES

Take the (nonprice) rationing of organ transplants, for example. Currently, in the United States no "market" exists for transplant organs. Donated organs are supposedly available on the basis of need. Yet, despite the existence of a nonprofit organ donor system that supposedly does not discriminate on ability to pay, the rate of organ transplantation among minorities is proportionally lower than for whites. According to the United Network for Organ Sharing, African Americans received only 3.7 percent of pancreases despite comprising 8 percent of those waiting. Blacks received only 14.9 percent of living donor kidneys and 27 percent of cadaveric kidneys despite comprising 34.8 percent of the people on the waiting list.[3]

Other evidence points to discrimination in the U.S. health care system. Many studies have found that ethnic minorities receive fewer routine services and lower-quality medical care than whites. The reasons include lower rates of health insurance coverage and the fact that minority patients sometimes wait longer to seek care. However, the disparities tend to narrow significantly—if not disappear altogether—when adjusted for income and other socioeconomic differences.[4]

By contrast, few studies of how racial minorities fare under national health insurance in other countries have been published. The few studies that exist, together with surveys and anecdotal evidence, are consistent with what economic theory would predict: minority patients do not fare well under nonprice rationing of health care.

RACIAL DISCRIMINATION IN BRITAIN

In Britain, uneven levels of access and treatment for the country's growing minority population (mostly South Asian) have fueled claims of racism within the NHS. For example, according to the British newspaper *The Guardian*, a confidential government report as well as an independent think tank report found racism flourishing in the NHS.[5] In one case, the NHS had accepted an organ donation for white patients only.[6]

A survey of GPs in England found diabetes and asthma programs were more common in affluent, mostly white areas than in inner-city London, which has a high minority population. The NHS also was less likely to equip hospitals in London's minority areas for cervical cancer testing and childhood immunization.[7]

RACIAL DISCRIMINATION IN CANADA

Similar problems have been identified with respect to indigenous minorities in Canada.[8] In a recent study of Canadian Indian groups, researchers found that all of the groups sampled had much less access to health care than Caucasians, despite their greater health needs. For example, the infant death rate during the study period was 13.8 per 1,000 live births for Indian infants and 16.3 per 1,000 for Inuit infants, approximately twice the rate (7.3 per 1,000) for all Canadian infants during the same period. Overall, Canadian aboriginal people "die earlier than their fellow Canadians and sustain a disproportionate share of the burden of physical disease and mental illness."[9]

RACIAL DISCRIMINATION IN NEW ZEALAND

In New Zealand, the average life expectancy for Maori men (sixty-eight years) is 5.5 years less than for non-Maori men, and six years less for Maori women (seventy-three years) than for non-Maori women.[10] Furthermore, those Maori who live in the least deprived areas live seven years longer than those in the most deprived areas. The corresponding figure for women is eight years. The disparities do not stop with life expectancy. Most diabetes is preventable (or manageable) through early diagnosis and intervention. However, its incidence among forty-five- to sixty-four-year-old Maori is four times that of comparable non-Maori. The incidence of high blood pressure among young (25–44) Maori men and women is almost twice the rates of non-Maori New Zealand men and women of European ancestry.[11]

RACIAL DISCRIMINATION IN AUSTRALIA

Australia also has a significant minority population (the Aborigines). Various studies have reported that[12]

- Aborigines are three times more likely to die in infancy than white Australians and about half of the survivors will die before they reach age fifty.
- Of all Aborigines who died between 1995 and 1997, 53 percent of men and 41 percent of women were under age fifty; by comparison, 13 percent of all other Australian men and 7 percent of all other Australian women who died were under age fifty. The disparities appear to be a result of health care access inequalities.
- Death rates are higher for Aborigines in all age groups. In infancy, Aborigines are 3.1 to 3.5 times more likely to die than other Australians. In the thirty-five to fifty-four age group, they are six to seven times more likely to die than other Australians.

Despite the greater overall health needs of these populations, minorities in countries with single-payer systems are routinely marginalized by systems that direct resources and services toward the more affluent, white, urban majority.

NOTES

1. For a discussion, see Michael Lowe, Ian H. Kerridge and Kenneth R Mitchell, "'These Sorts of People Don't Do Very Well': Race and Allocation of Health Care Resources," *Journal of Medical Ethics* 21, no. 6 (December 1995).

2. See Gary S. Becker, *The Economics of Discrimination*, 2nd ed. (Chicago: University of Chicago Press, 1971).

3. *2001 Annual Report of the U.S. Organ Procurement and Transplantation Network and the Scientific Registry for Transplant Recipients: Transplant Data 1991–2000*, U.S. Department of Health and Human Services, 2001, available at www.ustransplant.org. In 2000, blacks comprised 36 percent of those waiting for kidneys, and 8 percent of those waiting for a pancreas. Blacks do receive a proportionate number of donor hearts (13.4 percent) while comprising an identical proportion of those waiting (13.4 percent); see also G. Caleb Alexander and Ashwini R. Sehgal, "Barriers to Cadaveric Renal Transplantation among Blacks, Women and the Poor," *Journal of the American Medical Association* 280, no. 13 (October 7, 1998): 1148–52; John Z. Ayanian et al., "The Effect of Patients' Preferences on Racial Differences in Access to Renal Transplantation," *New England Journal of Medicine* 341, no. 22 (November 25, 1999): 1661–69.

4. Brian D. Smedley, Adrienne Y. Stith and Alan R. Nelson, eds., *Unequal Treatment: Confronting Racial and Ethnic Disparities in Health Care* (Washington, D.C.: National Academy Press, Institute of Medicine, March 2002).

5. John Carvel, "Secret Government Report Finds Racism Flourishing in NHS," *Guardian Unlimited*, June 25, 2001; Carvel, "NHS Staff Tell of Morale-Sapping Racism," *Guardian Unlimited*, June 25, 2001; Carvel, "Racism Is Rife in NHS, Says Study," *Guardian Unlimited,* June 19, 2001.

6. The incident took place in July 1998. Sarah Boseley, David Brindle and Vikram Dodd, "NHS Took Organs Donated for Whites Only," *Guardian Unlimited*, July 7, 1999; and Sarah Boseley, "Transplant Chief Loses Job over Racism Row," *Guardian Unlimited,* February 23, 2000. For a report on this event and the NHS policy, see "An Investigation into Conditional Organ Donation—The Report of the Panel," UK Department of Health, February 2000.

7. Brenda Leese and Nick Bosanquet, "Change in General Practice and Its Effects on Service Provision in Areas with Different Socioeconomic Characteristics," *British Medical Journal* 311, no. 7004 (August 26, 1995): 546–50.

8. Aboriginal people have less access to health care services than other Canadians because of geographic location and a shortage of personnel trained to meet their needs. See Harriet L. MacMillan et al., "Aboriginal Health," *Canadian Medical Association Journal* 155, no. 11 (December 1, 1996): 1569–78. Also see "CMA's Submission to the Royal Commission on Aboriginal Peoples," in *Bridging the Gap: Promoting Health and Healing for Aboriginal Peoples in Canada* (Ottawa: Canadian Medical Association, 1994), 9–17; *Aboriginal Health in Canada* (Ottawa: Medical Services Branch, Health Canada, 1994); and Vincent F. Tookenay, "Improving the Health Status of Aboriginal People in Canada: New Directions, New Responsibilities," *Canadian Medical Association Journal* 155, no. 11 (December 1, 1996): 1581–83.

9. MacMillan et al., "Aboriginal Health."

10. Lisa Macdonald, "Maori/Non-Maori Lives: The Widening Gap," *Green Left Weekly*, no. 326, (July 29, 1998), available at http://jinx.sistm.unsw.edu.au/~greenlft/1998/326/326p23b.htm; and Michele Grigg and Ben Macrae, *Tikanga Oranga Hauora* (Health Trends), Ministry of Maori Development, Wellington, New Zealand, Whaka-pakari No 4., 2000, available at www.tpk.govt.nz/maori/education/tohtrend.pdf.

11. Grigg and Macrae, *Tikanga Oranga Hauora.*

12. "The Health and Welfare of Australia's Aboriginal and Torres Strait Island Peoples," Australian Bureau of Statistics, 2000. For similar trends in health care for New Zealand's Maori population, see "Our Health, Our Future: The Health of New Zealanders 1999," New Zealand Ministry of Health, 1999, and "Maori Health," *Healthcare Review—Online* 2, no. 4, December 1997.

Chapter Seventeen

Rural Areas

MYTH NO. 17: SINGLE-PAYER NATIONAL HEALTH INSURANCE WOULD BENEFIT RESIDENTS OF RURAL AREAS

What we know about who gets care and who does not under nonprice rationing schemes is incomplete. However, geographical variations in health care resources and health care outcomes exist.[1] Despite extensive efforts to combat geographic disparities in access to medical services, Canada, Britain, New Zealand and Australia all have medically underserved areas.[2]

Waiting times are longer in rural areas, principally because advanced medical equipment is in short supply there. Such technology, which is expensive, is often available only at major hospitals in large cities. In addition, since care is given only to patients who are available when an opening occurs in the surgery schedule, rural patients are at a considerable logistical disadvantage. Urban patients, who live close to medical facilities, benefit most from public provision. Their rural counterparts often have to travel hundreds of miles just to receive treatment. So, in using waiting as a rationing device, public systems indirectly discriminate against rural patients.

Even in urban areas, as we have seen, success in obtaining care often depends on the politics of bureaucracy. A patient treated by a physician in a rural area will tend to be at a disadvantage vis-à-vis a patient represented by a physician who lives nearby and is a colleague of the hospital staff. Urban patients also have access to political and personal relationships that may be important in dealing with bureaucratic obstacles—relationships rural patients seldom have.

RURAL PATIENTS IN BRITAIN

Britain is one of the few countries that publishes hospital waiting lists by region and for the country as a whole. Yet, in Britain, as in other countries with single-payer systems, rationing decisions are made by doctors and hospital personnel at the local level. No national procedures guarantee that those in greater need move to the front of the waiting lines.

The most important philosophical principle set forth by those who established the British NHS was equal access to health care. Yet, as we noted above, inequalities across England persist and may even have grown worse since the NHS was founded in 1948. The British government tends to spend the most in metropolitan areas—especially the wealthier urban districts—where private sector alternatives are most abundant. For example, the NHS spends 20 percent of its annual budget on the greater London area, although the 15 percent of the population living there has access to the most private sector services. Nonetheless, there are persistent pleas to allocate even more resources to the London area.[3]

Overall, the quantities of resources allocated to different regions of the country are vastly different.[4]

- The North East Thames region (near London) has 27 percent more doctors and dentists per person, 15 percent more hospital beds and 12 percent more total health spending than the Trent region (in the more rural northern part of the country).
- There are 63 doctors per 100 beds at University College London Hospital Trust in London, compared to 11 doctors per 100 beds at the hospital in Northern Devon, a rural area in southern England.
- At Chelsea and Westminster Healthcare Trust, located in one of London's most prosperous districts, there are 64 doctors per 100 beds, compared to only 18 doctors per 100 beds at Pinderfields Hospital in rural West Yorkshire.

These differences in resources reinforce regional disparities in the levels of care patients receive. To be sure, government reforms of the past two decades have brought some noticeable declines in the waiting list numbers. However, it is significant to note that some areas have seen greater improvement than others. Table 17.1 shows changes in the waiting lists for the three best- and worst-performing health authorities in England:

- Between March 1997 and March 1999, the total number of patients waiting for medical treatment in the three London health authorities fell by between 23 and 31 percent.
- Over the same period, the total number of patients waiting for medical treatment in the three rural health authorities increased by between 12 and 19 percent.[5]

TABLE 17-1

Percentage Change in Number of Patients On Waiting Lists between March 1997 and March 1999 for London and Rural Areas

London Health Authorities	Percentage Change
Brent and Harrow	-23.4%
Croydon	-24.1%
Camden and Islington	-31.6%

Selected Rural Health Authorities	Percentage Change
South Staffordshire	+19.9%
Wocestershire	+12.9%
Warwickshire	+12.8%

Source: "Hospital Waiting List Statistics: England," *NHS Executive*, 2000.

For individual hospital trusts within London and rural health authorities, the differences in levels of treatment and health outcomes are even more striking.[6]

- At Homerton Hospital in London, 96 percent of inpatients are admitted within six months, compared to 51 percent of patients at Surrey and Sussex Healthcare Trust in the rural southeast.
- Similarly, at Whittington Hospital in London, 90 percent of inpatients are admitted within six months, compared to 54 percent of patients at Royal Surrey County Hospital in the rural southeast.

These inequalities do not reflect differences in need. Northerners die younger and are less healthy than southerners.[7] Poor urban dwellers live shorter lives and die more frequently from common, treatable illnesses than their wealthier neighbors living only blocks away. For example[8]:

- A person with colon cancer in Herefordshire has a 52.4 percent chance of survival, while a person in the rural northeastern town of Tees has a 24.9 percent chance.
- A woman with breast cancer living in the Hillingdon, Borough of London, has an 80.3 percent chance of surviving five years, compared to a 64.5 percent chance for a woman in rural North Staffordshire.

Clearly, peoples' chances of surviving major illnesses or procedures depend very much on where they live. Although some of the differences in outcomes may be attributable to regional differences in lifestyle, differences in medical resources must surely matter. The difference in cancer mortality and survival rates, for example, has been attributed to the general shortage of specialists, unavailability of the latest cancer drugs and relative lack of investment in radiotherapy equipment in underserved health regions.[9]

RURAL PATIENTS IN CANADA

In Canada, too, wide differences exist between the level of care available to citizens who live in the sparsely populated countryside and those who live in metropolitan areas. Although rural residents pay the same high tax rates as urban dwellers, they have less access to care. Recent hospital closings are a serious problem for rural patients. According to the *Canadian Journal of Rural Medicine,* "In Alberta, Saskatchewan and Manitoba rural hospitals have been closed by the dozens."[10]

Not surprisingly, the number of family physicians—as well as the number of specialists—varies widely across the rural and urban centers. In British Columbia, the average family physician in the rural Peace Liard region has 1,316 patients, while his counterpart in urban Vancouver has 606 patients. If specialists are included, there are 1,099 patients per physician in the Peace Liard region compared to 268 in Vancouver.[11] There are also inequalities among the provinces:

- Among Canadian provinces, the number of physicians per 100,000 population varies from a high of 211 in Quebec to a low of 92 in the Northwest Territories, a difference of more than 2 to 1.[12]
- The number of patient beds varies from a high of 22.3 per 1,000 population in Prince Edward Island to 10.6 per 1,000 in Yukon Territory, a difference of more than 2 to 1.[13]

As noted above, health care in Canada tends to be hospital-based, with modern technology restricted to teaching hospitals and outpatient surgery discouraged. Moreover, specialists and major hospitals tend to be in major cities. As in other countries, rural residents often travel to the larger cities for medical care. A major study produced at the University of British Columbia determined the impact this has on the amount of care urban and rural patients receive. As previously noted, this study is unique in that it identified patients based on where they lived and thus was able to accurately determine how much care was delivered to the population of the different health regions. Table 17.2 and figure 17.1 show the following:[14]

- Overall, people living in British Columbia's two largest cities (Vancouver and Victoria) received about 63 percent more physician services per capita than those living in the twenty-seven rural districts of the province.
- Urban residents received 91 percent more services from specialists per capita than rural residents, and for specific specialties the discrepancies were even greater.
- On the average, urban residents were seven times more likely to receive services from a thoracic surgeon, almost four times more likely to receive the services of a psychiatrist, almost three times more likely to receive services from a dermatologist and twice as likely to receive services from a neurologist.

TABLE 17-2

Spending on Physician Services
Per Person in British Columbia[1]
(1993-94)

Speciality	Urban[2]	Rural[3]	Urban/Rural
All Physician Services	$494.5	$303.0	163%
General Practice	173.2	142.3	122%
Specialists	321.3	168.5	191%
Anesthesia	30.0	9.6	313%
Dermatology	6.5	2.4	271%
General Surgery	15.9	13.8	115%
Internal Medicine	39.3	21.3	185%
Neurology	5.7	2.8	204%
Neurosurgery	2.5	1.3	192%
OB/GYN	13.5	8.6	157%
Ophthalmology	22.9	9.7	236%
Orthopedic Surgery	9.7	7.8	124%
Ontolaryngology	7.7	3.9	197%
Pediatrics	11.5	4.7	245%
Pathology	59.8	39.0	153%
Plastic Surgery	4.85	2.3	211%
Psychiatry	22.6	5.7	396%
Radiology	44.5	26.9	165%
Thoracic Surgery	7.1	1.0	710%
Urology	7.0	4.4	159%

[1] Based on fees paid to physicians for rendering services to patients living in the areas indicated, regardless of the area in which the service was performed. All figures are age-sex standardized and expressed in Canadian dollars.

[2] Greater Vancouver and Victoria regional hospital districts.

[3] Twenty-seven non-metropolitan hospital districts.

Source: Arminée Kazanjian et al., "Fee Practice Medical Expenditures per Capita and Full-Time Equivalent Physicians in British Columbia, 1993-94," University of British Columbia, Centre for Health Services and Policy Research, 1995.

FIGURE 17-1

Inequalities in the Use of
Physician Services among Urban and
Rural Patients in British Columbia
(Per capita spending, 1993-94)

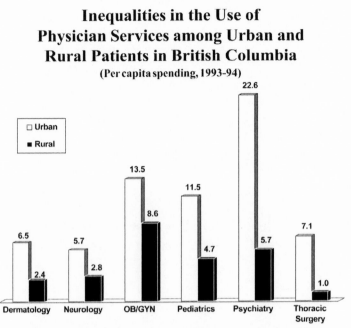

Sources: Arminée Kazanjian et al., "Fee Practice Medical Expenditures Per Capita and
Full-Time Equivalent Physicians in British Columbia, 1993-94," University of
British Columbia, 1995.

NOTES

1. Nigel Rice and Peter C. Smith, "Ethics and Geographical Equity in Health Care," *Journal of Medical Ethics* 27, no. 4 (August 2001), 256.

2. Morris L. Barer, Laura Wood and David G. Schneider, "Toward Improved Access to Medical Services for Relatively Underserved Populations: Canadian Approaches, Foreign Lessons," Centre for Health Services and Policy Research, University of British Columbia, May 1999.

3. Mike Pringle, "Primary Care: Opportunities and Threats. An Opportunity to Improve Primary Care," *British Medical Journal* 314, no. 7080 (February 22, 1997): 595–97.

4. "Good Hospital Guide for Britain and Ireland," Dr. Foster, 2001, cited in the *Sunday Times,* January 2001.

5. National Health Service, "Hospital Waiting List Statistics: England," *NHS Executive* (2000).

6. "Good Hospital Guide for Britain and Ireland," Dr. Foster, 2001.

7. "Dying of Inequality," *The Economist* (April 4, 1987): 52; see also "UK Death Rate Echoes North-South Divide," *Reuters Health,* 2000.

8. "Cancer Rates Reveal Regional Divide," *BBC News,* July 13, 2000; National Health Service, "NHS Postcode Lottery Revealed" and "Quality and Performance in the NHS. Performance Indicators: July 2000," *NHS Executive* (July 2000).

9. "Cancer Rates Reveal Regional Divide," *BBC News,* July 13, 2000.

10. John Wootton, "Rural Hospitals: We Can't Do without Them!" *Canadian Journal of Rural Medicine* 2, no. 2 (Spring 1997): 59.

11. Harvey V. Thommasen et al., "Physician: Population Ratios in British Columbia," *Canadian Journal of Rural Medicine* 4, no. 3 (Summer 1999): 139–45.

12. Southam Medical Database, Canadian Institute for Health Information, 2001.

13. "Health Care Beds, All Institutions, by Type of Care," Statistics Canada, Canadian Institute for Health Information, 1996–97, available at www.statcan.ca/english/Pgdb/People/Health/health32a.htm.

14. Arminée Kazanjian et al., "Fee Practice Medical Expenditures per Capita and Full-Time Equivalent Physicians in British Columbia, 1993–94," University of British Columbia, 1995. Physicians in Canada are paid by the province on a fee-for-service basis. Income data are available by specialty for each region. Consequently, fee-for-service income is a good measure of the value of services actually rendered to patients. By using physician billing data, the researchers determined the regional hospital district in which each patient lived—even if the service was provided in some other district.

Chapter Eighteen

Prescription Drugs

MYTH NO. 18: SINGLE-PAYER NATIONAL HEALTH INSURANCE WOULD REDUCE THE COST OF PRESCRIPTION DRUGS FOR AMERICANS

Advocates of single-payer insurance maintain that it would simultaneously: (1) provide all Americans with full coverage for necessary drugs and (2) contain drug costs. They say it would do so by establishing a national formulary—a list of drugs available to patients under the national health program—and by negotiating drug prices with manufacturers "based on their costs (excluding marketing or lobbying)."[1]

These ideas appeal to many Americans facing high prescription drug costs. However, access to new, more effective drugs is often restricted in countries with national health insurance. Furthermore, although some drugs cost less in other countries, other drugs cost more. Studies in the mid-1990s showed that U.S. prices were not necessarily higher than in other developed countries, nor was per capita spending on drugs. Recent updates of those studies show somewhat higher prices in the United States, but international prices are very similar, relative to average incomes. U.S. per capita spending now exceeds that of most other countries, but that may not be a bad development, especially if drug therapies are substituting for more expensive hospital and physician therapies. In fact, evidence suggests that at least for the elderly we may be spending too little on drugs.

WHY NEW DRUGS ARE SO COSTLY

Pharmaceutical companies that develop new drugs have an exclusive right for a limited number of years to manufacture their product under U.S. patent laws and international treaties. Patents allow drug makers to recoup their costs, and encourage companies to take the financial risk of drug development. Only one in five drugs tested ever reaches the market, making drug development very costly, now averaging about $900 million for each new drug.[2] Further, once patent protection has lapsed, any rival company can manufacture and sell a generic equivalent. At that point, the price of the generic tends to equal production costs alone, regardless of the original costs of development.

PRICE CONTROLS

We saw in chapter 13 that some advocates of single-payer national health insurance are envious of the ability of governments in other countries to exploit their monopsony bargaining power to push down the fees of doctors and other health workers. A similar principle applies to drugs. If manufacturers have to bargain with a single entity, acting on behalf of an entire country, they are at a severe disadvantage.

A government facing continual crises of rising health care costs is tempted to insist on prices just above the costs of production, ignoring all the R&D costs. Thus, the country could try to reap the benefits of new drugs without sharing in the expense of their development. When push comes to shove, pharmaceutical companies are tempted to give in to such demands, since the development costs are sunk costs. They may conclude that as long as they cover the costs of production, something is better than nothing.

However, if every country in the world were to follow this strategy and succeed, no one would be left to pay for R&D. That means no new drugs. Some policies that seem smart from a purely local point of view can have disastrous consequences internationally. Politicians in other countries want the United States to pay all the development costs while they reap the benefits. Single-payer advocates in this country overlook the fact that if the United States followed the same strategy, there would be no one left to pay for R&D.

Countries with less money to reinvest in R&D have seen their pharmaceutical industries decline or go abroad. The United States, which has no widespread price controls, produces far more drug innovations than any other country.

DO EUROPEANS HAVE ACCESS
TO THE SAME DRUGS AS AMERICANS?

One way OECD countries control drug expenditures is by delaying the market-place introduction of the newest drugs or by restricting access to them. To speed access to new drugs, the European Union took steps to centralize the process for marketing authorization through the European Agency for the Evaluation of Medicines in 1995. However, drug companies must go through additional steps in order to make their drugs available to patients. After a drug is approved by the EU, drug makers must negotiate the selling price with each national government. And, finally, they separately negotiate the "reimbursement rate," or subsidy, provided by the EU to the drug companies for important new drugs. Until all these hurdles are cleared, new drugs are unavailable to most patients.[3]

Because of these barriers to entry, patients in some European countries wait months or even years longer than patients in America for access to new medications, including breakthrough drugs. For instance, according to studies by Europe Economics, a London-based research organization,[4]

- A major new medication that treats the nervous system was not accessible to patients for three additional years in France and nearly six years in Portugal after its introduction in the United States.
- An important new anti-infection therapy already available in other EU countries was not accessible to patients for three years in Belgium and France and for more than four years in Portugal and Greece.
- A new cardiovascular drug available in other EU countries was withheld for almost three years from patients in Portugal, Spain and Greece.

ACCESS TO DRUGS IN BRITAIN

In Britain, many drugs that are available to private pay patients are not available to NHS patients. Each local health authority can decide which drugs are placed on its formulary, and due to budget limitations, expensive drugs are often left off the lists. As a result, NHS patients are often denied the best drug therapy. For example:

- Dr. Edward Newlands, the British doctor who codeveloped the brain cancer drug Temodal, cannot prescribe it to his patients.[5]
- Taxol, a drug that is widely prescribed in the United States for the treatment of breast cancer, and Gemzar, a drug used to treat pancreatic cancer, are unavailable in some regions of the United Kingdom.[6]

• Fewer than one-third of British patients who suffer a heart attack have access to beta-blockers used by 75 percent of patients in the United States, despite the fact that post-heart attack use of the drug reduces the risk of sudden death from a subsequent heart attack by 20 percent.[7]

Recall also the conclusion of a WHO study that lack of access to the best cancer drugs costs the lives of 25,000 Britons every year.[8]

ACCESS TO DRUGS IN CANADA

In recent years the news media have featured stories about buses heading to Canada loaded with Americans in search of cheaper Canadian drugs.[9] What many people may not have heard is that some Canadians travel to the United States to buy drugs not available at any price in Canada. For example, one of the newest drugs to treat noninsulin dependent diabetes—Glucophage XR— is not available in Canada.[10] Canada tries to control drug costs through price controls and provincial formularies. Manufacturers are allowed to charge higher prices for new drugs that the federal Patented Medicines Price Review Board decides are a substantial improvement over existing drugs. Of the 581 drugs reviewed between 1988 and 1995, only 41 were allowed to earn a higher return.[11] From 1994 through 1998 the board approved only 24 of the 400 drugs considered, ruling that the rest were not substantial improvements over their predecessors.[12]

In addition, each of Canada's ten provinces has a review committee that must approve the drug for that province's formulary, which determines which drugs will be paid by the health program. A drug may be approved by one province, but not another. For instance, of the twenty-three cardiovascular drugs approved by the national government between 1991 and 1998, one province covered only ten while another covered twenty-three.[13]

Approval times for additions to formularies vary greatly from province to province. For instance, while Nova Scotia approves drugs for its formulary in 250 days, it takes nearly 500 days in Ontario.[14] In theory, Canadians can buy any federally approved drug, even if it is not on the provincial formulary, by paying for it themselves. However, drug companies often don't market those drugs widely because the demand is so low.[15]

A University of Toronto study concluded that the main effect of price controls has been to limit patients' choices, causing them to rely more on hospitals and surgery.[16] British Columbia has gone farther than most provinces in controlling access to new drugs. Under its "reference price system" it can require that a patient receiving subsidized drugs under the provincial health program be treated with the least costly drug, even if it is a completely different compound, as long as it is deemed to have the same therapeutic effect. Since the effectiveness and side effects of drugs vary from patient to patient, frequent therapeutic substitution has harmed patients.[17]

- 27 percent of physicians in British Columbia report that they have had to admit patients to the emergency room or hospital as a result of the mandated switching of medicines.
- 68 percent report confusion or uncertainty in cardiovascular or hypertension patients, and 60 percent have seen patients' conditions worsen or their symptoms accelerate due to mandated switching.

Dr. William McArthur, former chief coroner for British Columbia, recalls from his own practice a sixty-four-year-old male patient who had controlled peptic ulcers for more than five years. When the government required that he be switched to an older, less effective drug, within three days he required hospitalization and a lifesaving blood transfusion. After ten days in the hospital and several more transfusions, he was discharged and placed on the drug he had taken originally.[18]

ARE PRESCRIPTION DRUG PRICES LOWER IN OTHER COUNTRIES?

Comparing prices across countries is complicated. Pharmaceutical companies, like makers of other products, charge different prices in different countries. In the United States, the list prices of drugs are generally used as reference points for calculating discounts and are not usually the price actually paid. Also, the top-selling drugs in one country are not the top sellers in others, so one cannot simply compare top sellers. Further, generic drugs often have higher volumes and lower prices than brand-name drugs.

Economist Patricia Danzon examined some well-publicized international price comparisons of pharmaceuticals and concluded that their findings of very large price differences between the United States and other industrial countries were based on flawed methodology. Among the errors: using small, nonrandom samples of products, excluding generic drugs (which make up 42 percent of U.S. purchases), ignoring differences in prescription and consumption patterns from country to country, and ignoring manufacturer discounts and rebates in the United States.[19]

Professor Danzon conducted her own comparison, attempting to control for all these complicating factors. She determined the manufacturers' prices for both brand-name drugs covered by patents and generic drugs in the United States and eight other countries, and converted the weights of each product to U.S. measures. Depending on the country and the drugs available, she compared from 187 to 484 products. She found that average prices of prescription drugs were comparable to or higher than U.S. prices in Canada, Germany, Sweden and Switzerland, and lower in France, Italy, Japan and the United Kingdom.[20]

More recent research by Danzon found that due to the recent weakness of the Canadian dollar, the relative prices of Canadian medications fell compared to the United States. Further, drug prices in Italy, Britain and Germany were approximately 15 percent lower (or less) than in the United States while prices in France and Canada were about 33 and 30 percent lower, respectively. However, for most countries, the prices charged reflect differences in living standards and national income. When these variations are taken into account drugs cost less in the United States than in the other countries surveyed, except in France.[21]

HOW SUCCESSFUL ARE PRICE CONTROLS AT HOLDING DOWN DRUG SPENDING?

Apparently not very, despite the fact that countries with single-payer systems try to limit both price and availability. OECD data from 1992 showed that when per capita spending on medications was adjusted for differences in the value of currency from country to country ("purchasing power parity"), the United States spent less than France, Germany and Japan. It spent a few dollars more than Canada and substantially more than Britain. More recently, spending in the United States has inched up relative to other countries, possibly because managed care organizations seized opportunities to substitute drug therapies for more expensive doctor and hospital therapies during the 1990s. Figure 18.1 shows the following:

- France spent $290 per capita on prescription drugs each year, compared to $283 for the United States.
- Spending in Japan ($281) was only slightly less than in the United States.
- Trailing these countries were Germany ($255), Canada ($237) and Britain ($162).

Note that if the greater U.S. spending in the 1990s is a result of the substitution of drug therapies for more expensive ones, this change represents an increase in efficiency.

FIGURE 18-1

A Comparison of Pharmaceutical Expenditures per Capita

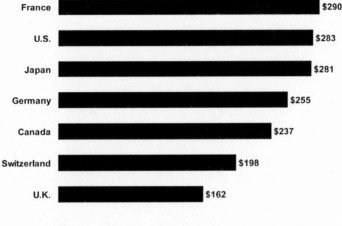

Note: Based on purchasing power parity, U.S. dollars. Data are for 1997.
Pharmaceuticals include nonprescription products.

Source: *OECD Health Data, 2002.*

DOES PRESCRIPTION DRUG SPENDING SAVE MONEY?

Despite its high cost, we are getting quite a bit of value for our investment in drugs. Drug therapy is one of the most efficient methods of treating disease. In many cases, drug therapies have reduced the cost of other health care services. Even greater savings are possible because in many cases newer drugs are more effective than older, less expensive drugs.

Research by Columbia University professor Frank Lichtenberg indicates that each dollar spent on drugs is associated with roughly a four-dollar decline in spending on hospitals.[22] Furthermore, a reduction in the age of drugs (substituting newer for older drugs) reduces spending on hospitalizations and doctor visits by 7.2 times as much as it increases drug expenditure. The number of hospital stays, bed days and surgical procedures declines most rapidly for those diagnoses with the greatest increase in the total number of drugs prescribed and the greatest use of new drugs.[23]

Overall, Lichtenburg's estimates imply that an increase of 100 prescriptions is associated with 1.48 fewer hospital admissions, 16.3 fewer hospital days and 3.36 fewer inpatient surgical procedures. He also estimates that new drugs have increased life expectancy by as much as 1 percent per year.[24]

SHOPPING FOR DRUGS

Patients whose drugs are paid for by a third party (a private insurer or government) have little incentive to shop for the best price. This is especially true in countries with controlled drug prices, where there is no price competition. American consumers, however, can significantly lower their drug costs by comparison shopping among American pharmacies, buying medications in large quantities and splitting double-dose pills.[25]

Using these techniques, in many cases patients can obtain drugs at lower prices in the United States than they could by purchasing them in Canada. For example, the *New York Times* compared U.S. and Canadian prices of ten drugs widely used by seniors. They found in all ten cases Canadian prices were lower. But they didn't look very far, and they didn't investigate shopping techniques that would be normal for any other consumer purchase. The National Center for Policy Analysis compared the Canadian price to the best price consumers could obtain using smart-shopping techniques. Table 18.1 shows the following:

- For seven of ten drugs, U.S. buyers can lower their costs an average of 38 percent below the price charged in Canada.
- For all ten drugs combined, smart buying in the U.S. produces an average cost of 10 percent below buying in Canada.

TABLE 18-1

U.S. Smart Shopping Versus Canada

Drug	Condition	Dose	Qt.	Best Canadian Price	Smart Shopping Cost	Smart Shopping Saving
Lipitor	High cholesterol	20mg	30	$60.66	$45.00	26%
Norvasc	High blood pressure	10mg	90	$153.66	$167.32	-9%
Paxil	Depression	20mg	30	$57.20	$40.86	29%
Premarin	Osteoporosis	0.625mg	100	$25.75	$77.90	-203%
Prevacid	Ulcers	30mg	30	$69.63	$21.42	69%
Synthroid	Hypothyroidism	0.05mg	100	$19.77	$10.83	45%
Toprol-XL	High blood pressure	100mg	90	$35.51	$17.00	52%
Zithromax	Antibiotic	250mg	6	$31.38	$41.95	-34%
Zocor	High cholesterol	20mg	30	$67.43	$54.30	19%
Zoloft	Depression	50mg	30	$45.54	$33.33	27%

Note: Based on National Center for Policy Analysis survey of pharmacy Web sites in Canada and the United States conducted in July 2003.

NOTES

1. Marcia Angell et al., Physicians' Working Group on Single-Payer National Health Insurance, "Proposal for Health Care Reform," Presentation to the Congressional Black Caucus and the Congressional Progressive Caucus, May 1, 2001.

2. Press Release, "Total Cost to Develop a New Prescription Drug, Including Cost of Post-Approval Research, Is $897 Million," May 13, 2003, Tufts Center for the Study of Drug Development, available at http://155.212.10.127/NewsEvents/RecentNews.asp? newsid=29, accessed December 15, 2003.

3. "In Europe, Access to New Medications Takes Time," Galen Institute, Alexandria, Va., September 28, 2000.

4. "Patient Access to Major Pharmaceutical Products in EU Member States," Europe Economics, 1998, and "Patient Access to Pharmaceuticals Approved through Mutual Recognition," Europe Economics, 1999, both cited in "In Europe, Access to New Medications Takes Time," Galen Institute, Alexandria, Va., September 28, 2000.

5. Grace-Marie Turner, "Foreign Countries Limit Access to Prescription Drugs," Galen Institute, Galen Reports, May 27, 2000, available at www.galen.org/news/052700 .html.

6. D. Taylor and J. Mossman, "Living with Ovarian Cancer," *CancerBACUP,* Care Survey, 1999; and "Is NICE Removing Postcode Prescribing?" *CancerBACUP,* November 2000.

7. See Neil C. Campbell et al., "Secondary Prevention in Coronary Heart Disease: Baseline Survey of Provision in General Practice," *British Medical Journal* 316, no. 7142 (May 9, 1998): 1430–34; and K. W. Clarke, D. Gray and J. R. Hampton, "Evidence of Inadequate Investigation and Treatment of Patients with Heart Failure," *British Heart Journal* 71, no. 6 (June 1994): 584–87. In the United States, a newer class of drugs is now replacing beta-blockers.

8. Karol Sikora, "Cancer Survival in Britain," *British Medical Journal* 319, no. 7208 (August 21, 1999), 461–62.

9. Karen Dandurant, "Seniors' Field Trip to Canada Saves Them $17K in Prescription Costs," *Portsmouth Herald*, November 8, 2003.

10. Merrill Matthews Jr., "On a Bus to Bangor, Canadians Seeking Health Care," *Wall Street Journal*, July 5, 2002.

11. Devidas Menon, "Pharmaceutical Cost Control in Canada: Does It Work?" *Health Affairs* 20, no. 3 (May/June 2001): 99.

12. William McArthur, "Prescription Drug Costs: Has Canada Found the Answer?" National Center for Policy Analysis, NCPA Brief Analysis No. 323, May 19, 2003.

13. Menon, "Pharmaceutical Cost Control."

14. McArthur, "Prescription Drug Costs."

15. Menon, "Pharmaceutical Cost Control," 100.

16. William McArthur, "Canadian Health Care—A System in Collapse," *Backgrounder*, Fraser Institute (January 27, 2000).

17. McArthur, "Canadian Health Care."

18. McArthur, "Canadian Health Care."

19. See Patricia M. Danzon, "The Uses and Abuses of International Price Comparisons," in *Competitive Strategies in the Pharmaceutical Industry*, R. B. Helms, ed. (Washington, D.C.: American Enterprise Institute Press, 1996); Patricia M. Danzon, *Pharmaceutical Price Regulation: National Policies Versus Global Interests* (Washington, D.C.: American Enterprise Institute Press, 1997); and Patricia M. Danzon and J. D. Kim, "The Life Cycle of Pharmaceuticals: A Cross-National Perspective," Wharton School, Wharton Working Paper, 1997.

20. Danzon, "The Uses and Abuses."

21. Patricia M. Danzon and Michael F. Furukawa, "Prices and Availability of Pharmaceuticals: Evidence from Nine Countries," *Health Affairs* (October 29, 2003) (Web exclusive). Countries surveyed were Canada, Chile, France, Germany, Italy, Japan, Mexico, the United Kingdom and the United States.

22. Frank Lichtenberg, "The Effect of Pharmaceutical Utilization and Innovation on Hospitalization and Mortality," National Bureau of Economic Research, Paper No. 5418, January 1996. Also, see Frank Lichtenberg, "Pharmaceutical Innovation, Mortality Reduction and Economic Growth," National Bureau of Economic Research, NBER Working Paper W6569, May 1998.

23. Frank Lichtenberg, "Benefits and Costs of Newer Drugs: An Update," National Bureau of Economic Research, NBER Working Paper W8996, June 2002.

24. Frank Lichtenberg, "Pharmaceutical Innovation, Mortality Reduction and Economic Growth," National Bureau of Economic Research, NBER Working Paper W6569, May 1998.

25. Devon M. Herrick, "Shopping for Drugs," National Center for Policy Analysis, Policy Report No. 262, June 2003.

Chapter Nineteen

Public Opinion

MYTH NO. 19: SINGLE-PAYER NATIONAL HEALTH INSURANCE WOULD BE POPULAR IN THE UNITED STATES

This notion is based largely on the assumption that what is popular in other countries would be popular here. However, although there is hardly a clamor in other countries to implement an American-style system, their health systems are less popular than they used to be and in some cases much less popular. For example, the proportion of Canadians satisfied with their health care system dropped from 56 percent to 20 percent between 1987 and 1997.[1] In Britain, the sad state of the NHS was a major issue in the last national election, with both conservative and labor parties decrying the long waits, low standards of care and even outright abuse reported in the British press. As figure 19.1 shows, it appears that people almost everywhere believe their health care system needs to be reformed, regardless of the system under which they live.[2]

AMERICAN POLLING RESULTS

Pollsters have long known that they can get different answers depending on how they phrase their questions. According to one set of polling results, most Americans are satisfied with their family's health care, although negative opinions about managed care are widespread.[3] As figure 19.2 shows, only about one-third of the U.S. public supports a complete overhaul of the system, including only 41 percent of the uninsured. Figure 19.2 shows that the proportion of Americans who are completely dissatisfied with the "accessibility and

FIGURE 19-1

Percent Who Agree with Statement:
Only "Minor" Changes Needed

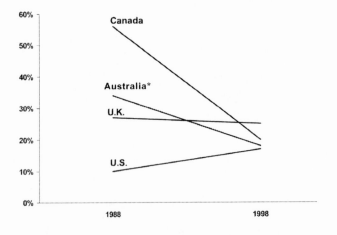

* 1990 data

Sources: Harvard/Harris/Baxter Survey, 1988 (Canada. U.K. and U.S.); Harvard,
Institute for the Future, 1990 (Australia); and Commonwealth Fund 1998
International Health Policy Survey.

FIGURE 19-2

Public Attitudes toward the U.S. Health Care System
(percent saying there is so much wrong it needs to be rebuilt)

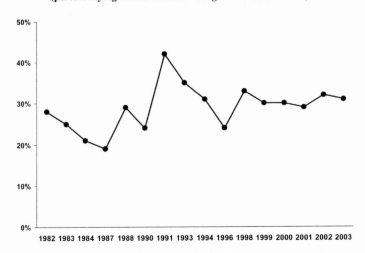

Source: Harris Interactive Polls, 1982-2003. Robert J. Blendon, "Americans' Views
on Health Care Policy," Harvard School of Public Health/Kennedy School
of Government, Harvard University (powerpoint presentation), September
2003.

affordability of health care" is substantially lower now than in 1993, when an overhaul of the health care system was proposed by President Clinton.[4]

These results appear to be contradicted by periodic surveys that find a majority of Americans favor a national health insurance program.[5] Indeed, as far back as the presidency of Richard Nixon, polls showed as much as 61 percent of the people favored it.[6] However, these polls frequently give no indication of what people are willing to give up for such a system—in terms of their willingness to pay higher taxes or to have their own health care rationed by government.[7] When surveys ask about taxes or rationing, support shrinks drastically. For instance, an analysis by the Harvard School of Public Health of a national poll taken in May through June 2003 found that less than half favored raising taxes to provide health insurance for all Americans.[8]

The initial question on a recent *Washington Post*-ABC News health care poll found that 62 percent of respondents favor a universal health care program run by the government and financed by taxpayers.[9] Some 79 percent thought that health insurance coverage for all Americans is important even if that means raising taxes. However, when asked if they would support universal health care if their choice of doctors were limited, 40 percent of those who had supported it changed their mind and opposed such a system. When asked if they would support universal health care with waiting lines for nonemergency treatment, support fell more than one-third, from 62 percent to 38 percent. Furthermore, 79 percent were opposed to the rationing of health care where an "increasing number of medical treatments that currently are covered by insurance will no longer be covered because they are too costly, not essential or have too little chance of success."

Even if socialized medicine were as popular with people who live under it as it is with advocates in this country, it would be unlikely to gain wide acceptance in the United States for one important reason: Americans are accustomed to a level of health care that single-payer national health insurance cannot provide. Precisely because the U.S. medical market is largely private, the vast majority of Americans are aware of advanced medical technology and have come to expect access to lifesaving equipment and procedures. Having witnessed the efficacy of private medicine, Americans are conditioned to expect immediate delivery of the best that medical science has to offer.

"Don't push me around" is a distinctively American phrase. In the United States we have widespread access to information about modern medical technology. In the age of the Internet, people are demanding more—not less—control over their health care.[10] We also have a legal system that protects the rights of those without political power or money and a strong devotion to basic rights of due process. Single-payer national health insurance, as it operates in other countries, simply would not survive in this country, given American culture and the U.S. legal system.

INFORMED HEALTH CARE CONSUMERS

Virtually all Americans have access to the Internet, and Web sites offering health information are among the most popular.[11] Approximately 15,000 to 20,000 Web sites deliver information on health and medicine.[12] In 1997, the National Library of Medicine moved away from a pay-per-use fee structure for its own "Medline" medical information Web site to one that is completely free.[13] Prior to this decision, Medline processed about seven million searches a year. In the first two years it was available on the Web for free, the number of Medline searches skyrocketed to 180 million a year, and the general public was performing a third of these searches.[14]

Americans also receive more health information through the mass media than do citizens of any other developed country. In August 1997, the U.S. Food and Drug Administration began allowing pharmaceutical companies to advertise prescription drugs on radio and television and in print without a lengthy summary of potential side effects and contraindications.[15] However, print advertising reproduces the detailed informational inserts that are included in drug packaging, including the health effects of the product. Television and radio commercials repeat health warnings about the most common side effects and the most at-risk populations.[16]

The FDA allows drug makers to make limited health claims for their products. In addition to manufacturers of drugs still under patent, aspirin makers, for example, disseminate information on regular aspirin use to prevent heart attacks and strokes.

This direct-to-consumer advertising bypasses physicians as gatekeepers of medical knowledge. Consumer knowledge of the existence and potential benefits of drugs increases their demand for those products.[17] Unsurprisingly, some physician groups oppose such advertising—since patients are less likely to put their complete trust in the decisions of health professionals if they are knowledgeable. By contrast, they are unlikely to demand alternative treatments if they are ignorant.

It is no coincidence that countries with national health insurance systems seek to ban such advertising.[18] Consumer awareness increases the cost of prescription drug programs.[19] Patients are less likely to be content if they know that they are denied access to newer, potentially more effective therapies because of cost-containing limits enforced through the health system's drug formulary.

NOTES

1. "Health Care in Canada 2000: A First Annual Report," Canadian Institute for Health Information, April 2000; cited in David Spurgeon, "Canadians Become Dissatisfied with Their Healthcare System," *British Medical Journal* 320, no. 7245 (May 13, 2000): 1295.

2. Commonwealth Fund 1998 International Health Policy Survey, cited in Karen Donelan et al., "The Cost of Health System Change: Public Discontent in Five Nations," *Health Affairs* 18, no. 3 (May/June 1999, Exhibit 6): 206–16.

3. Gary Langer, "Conflicting Views on HMOs," *ABCNEWS.com,* January 22, 1999.

4. Harris Interactive Polls, 1982–2003. Robert J. Blendon, "Americans' Views on Health Care Policy," Harvard School of Public Health/Kennedy School of Government, Harvard University (PowerPoint presentation), September 2003.

5. Bridget Harrison, "Historical Survey of National Health Movements and Public Opinion in the United States," *Journal of the American Medical Association* 289 (2003): 1163–64.

6. Jon Gabel, Howard Cohen and Steven Fink, "Americans' Views on Health Care: Foolish Inconsistencies?" *Health Affairs* 8, no. 1 (Spring 1989): 111.

7. Robert Weissberg, "Why Policymakers Should Ignore Public Opinion Polls," Cato Institute, Policy Analysis No. 402, May 29, 2001.

8. Press Release, "Problem of Uninsured Still Troubles Most Americans but Raising Taxes Remains a Sticking Point," *Health Affairs* (August 27, 2003).

9. "Washington Post–ABC News Poll: Health Care," *Washington Post*, October 20, 2003.

10. See Devon Herrick, "Managing Health Care with the Internet," National Center for Policy Analysis, Brief Analysis No. 330, July 27, 2000, and Devon Herrick, "Patient Power and the Internet," National Center for Policy Analysis, Brief Analysis No. 317, March 31, 2000.

11. Herrick, "Managing Health Care with the Internet."

12. Estimate by Bob Pringle, former president and cofounder of the health Web site Inteli-health, cited in Robert McGarvey, "Online Health's Plague of Riches," *Tech Insider* (September 29, 1999).

13. Joan Stephenson, "National Library of Medicine to Help Consumers Use Online Health Data," *Journal of the American Medical Association* 283, no. 13 (April 15, 2000): 1675–76.

14. Leslie Miller, "Guidelines Offer Cures for Web Confusion." *USA Today,* July 15, 1999.

15. Phyllis Maguire, "How Direct-to-Consumer Advertising Is Putting the Squeeze on Physicians," *ACP-ASIM Observer,* American College of Physicians–American Society of Internal Medicine, March 1999.

16. To read a longer review of regulations concerning direct-to-consumer advertising of pharmaceuticals, see Michie Hunt, "Direct-to-Consumer Advertising of Prescription Drugs," National Health Policy Forum, April 1998.

17. Barbara Mintzes, "Influence of Direct to Consumer Pharmaceutical Advertising and Patients' Requests on Prescribing Decisions: Two-Site Cross-Sectional Survey," *British Medical Journal* 324, no. 7332 (February 2, 2002), 278–79.

18. The United States and New Zealand were the only developed countries that allowed direct-to-consumer advertising as of March 2003. Bob Burton, "Ban Direct to Consumer Advertising, Report Recommends," *British Medical Journal* 326, no. 7387 (March 1, 2003), 467. Three-quarters of New Zealand physicians surveyed said that patients frequently asked for advertised drugs they did not consider appropriate, and only 12 percent of the doctors thought advertising was useful in educating patients. The European Commission had proposed to allow limited direct-to-consumer advertising of medications for certain conditions such as AIDS, asthma and diabetes, but EU health ministers rejected the proposal.

19. By one estimate, it would add C$1.2 billion to drug spending in Canada. Barbara Mintzes et al., "How Does Direct-to-Consumer Advertising (DTCA) Affect Prescribing? A Survey in Primary Care Environments with and without Legal DTCA," *Canadian Medical Association Journal* 169, no. 5 (September 2, 2003): 405–12.

Chapter Twenty

Reform

MYTH NO. 20: ADOPTING THE HEALTH CARE PROGRAMS OF OTHER COUNTRIES REQUIRES GOVERNMENT

Some of the proponents of national health insurance are leaders from industries that experience high health care costs and must compete with firms from countries with national health insurance. These leaders complain high health care costs make their industries less competitive compared to nationalized systems found in other countries.

The chairman of Ford Motor Company, William Clay Ford Jr., has stated that for automakers, health care cost is the "biggest issue on our plate that we can't solve."[1] Also, the U.S. president of the United Auto Workers, Ron Gettelfinger, is a proponent of a "universal, comprehensive, single-payer health-care program to cover every man, woman and child in the United States." This is not the first time auto workers and auto makers have looked longingly at the health care systems of other countries and called for a government solution. Nearly a decade ago Chrysler Chairman Lee Iacocca complained "about the great imbalance between health care costs in the United States and national health care systems in virtually every other country."[2] But do the workers at Chrysler and Ford really need government in order to adopt the health care programs of other countries? It is not at all clear that they do.

As we have seen, the primary way other developed countries control health care costs is through "global budgets." Hospitals, physicians or area health authorities are told by government how much money they have to spend. The government then leaves decisions about how to ration the funds to the health care bureaucracy.[3]

There is nothing mysterious about this process, and no reason why Chrysler and Ford need government in order to copy it. For example, auto workers or any other large group could form their own national health insurance plan. The total amount of money given to the national health insurance plan each year could be 75 percent or even 50 percent of what Chrysler or Ford now spends on employee health care, and the national health insurance plan managers could be instructed to ration care to their respective employees.

If Chrysler or Ford workers wanted to exert more direct control, they could elect the chief executive officer of the national health insurance plan in annual balloting, and the candidacy could be open to all health care bureaucrats or restricted to those with certain qualifications. The most obvious obstacle automakers would face would be U.S. tort law. If the national health insurance plan physicians rationed medical care the way the British do, there would be many potential malpractice suits. But if autoworkers owned their own HMO and if enough legal documents were signed, even this obstacle might be surmountable.

In short, Chrysler and Ford employees could realize "benefits" of national health insurance through private action, without government intervention, provided that is their sincere objective. On the other hand, if the rhetoric coming from automakers is merely a ruse to get taxpayers to pay autoworkers' annual health care bill, federal government coercion would be required.

A similar principle holds true for cities, states and other entities. Any organization that truly wishes to enjoy the benefits of a system of health insurance based on waiting lines, fixed budgets and rationed services could adopt many of the same principles used in Canada and Britain. For instance, a city government might allocate a fixed amount of funds to meet the health needs of its employees and their families and every other local citizen who elects to join as well. It could also empower a bureaucracy to ration health services. Those unable to obtain immediate care might be placed in a queue and receive care at a later date, possibly the following year. In allocating medical resources in this manner, the city might not meet all the needs of all its enrollees, but at least the national health insurance plan's spending would be lower, say, than what a Blue Cross plan would cost.

Although this arrangement is possible, it is doubtful city employees would tolerate it for long, however.

NOTES

1. Quentin Young, "National Health Insurance is the Obvious Prescription," *Chicago Tribune*, June 29, 2003.

2. Employee Benefits Research Institute, "EBRI Notes," *Employee Benefits Research Institute* 14, no. 2 (February 1993).

3. See the discussion in Jönsson, "What Can Americans Learn from Europeans?" 84–86.

Part Two

THE POLITICS AND ECONOMICS OF HEALTH CARE SYSTEMS

Chapter Twenty-one

The Politics of Medicine

"Public choice" is the discipline that attempts to integrate economics and political science.[1] Its chief goal is to explain political phenomena, just as economists explain purely economic phenomena. The name, however, is potentially misleading. The new discipline could more accurately be called "modern political science."

A fascinating discovery of this discipline is that economic principles, if carefully applied, explain much of what happens in politics. Take the concept of competition. Just as producers of goods and services compete for consumer dollars, so politicians in a democracy compete for votes. Moreover, the process of competition leads to certain well-defined results.

In the economic marketplace, competition inevitably forces producers to choose the most efficient method of production. Those who fail to do so either go out of business or mend their ways. The outcome—efficient production—is independent of any particular producer's wishes or desires.

In a similar way, political competition inexorably leads candidates to adopt specific positions, called the winning platform.[2] The idea of a winning platform is a fairly simple one. It is a set of political policies that can defeat any other set of policies in an election. Politicians who want to be elected or re-elected have every incentive to endorse the winning platform. If they do not, they become vulnerable; for if their opponents adopt the winning platform and they do not, the opponents will win.

Of course in the real world, things are rarely so simple. Many factors influence voters other than substantive political issues—a candidate's religion, ethnicity, gender, general appearance, speaking ability, party affiliation, and so forth. Even when voters are influenced by real political issues, politicians do not always know what the winning platform is. Often they must guess at it. Nonetheless, public choice theory holds that, other things being equal, a candidate always improves his chances of winning by endorsing the winning platform. Hence, all candidates have an incentive to identify and endorse this platform.

This line of reasoning leads to the conclusion that in democratic systems with two major political parties, both tend to adopt the same policies. They do so not because the party leaders think alike or share the same ideological preferences, but because their top priority is to win elections and hold office.

Two corollaries follow from this conclusion. The first is that it is absurd to complain about the fact that "major candidates all sound alike" or that "it doesn't seem to make any difference who wins." The complaints are merely evidence that political competition is working precisely as the theory predicts. Indeed, the more accurate information political candidates receive through better polling techniques and computerization, the more similar they will become. The theory predicts that, in a world of perfect information, the policies of the two major parties would be identical.

The second corollary is more relevant to our purposes. In its extreme form, the corollary asserts that "politicians don't matter." Over the long haul, if we want to explain why we have the political policies we have, it is futile to investigate the motives, personalities and characters of those who hold office. Instead, we must focus on those factors that determine the nature of the winning platform.

This corollary is crucial to understanding single-payer health insurance. A great many British health economists who support socialized medicine are quick to concede that the British NHS has defects. But these defects, in their view, are not those of socialism; they merely represent a failure of political will or of the politicians in office. The ultimate goal, they hold, is to retain the system of socialized medicine and make it work better.

By contrast, we argue that the defects of single-payer health insurance systems are inevitable consequences of placing the market for health under the control of politicians. It is not true that British health care policy just happens to be as it is. Enoch Powell, a former minister of health who ran the British NHS, seems to have appreciated this insight. Powell wrote that "whatever is entrusted to politicians becomes political even if it is not political anyhow,"[3] and he went on to say that

The phenomena of Medicine and Politics . . . result automatically and necessarily from the nationalization of medical care and its provision gratis at the point of consumption. . . . These phenomena are implicit in such an organization and are not the accidental or incidental results of blemishes which can be "reformed" away while leaving the system as such intact.[4]

An extensive analysis of the British health care system shows that all of the major features of national health insurance can be explained in terms of public choice theory.[5] That is, far from being the consequence of preferences of politicians (who could be replaced by different politicians with different preferences in the next election), the major features of single-payer systems of national health insurance follow inevitably from the fact that politicians have the authority to allocate health care resources, and from that fact alone. The following is a brief summary.

THE AMOUNT OF SPENDING ON HEALTH SERVICES

One argument used to justify national health insurance is that, left to their own devices, individuals will not spend as much as they ought to spend on health care. This was a major reason why many middle- and upper-middle-class British citizens supported national health insurance for the working class. It was also a major reason why they supported formation of the NHS in 1948.[6] Many expected that, under socialized medical care, more total dollars would be spent on health care than would otherwise have been the case.

Yet, it is not clear that socialized medicine in Britain has increased overall spending on health care. It may even have had the opposite result. This was the contention of Dennis Lees, professor of economics at the University of Nottingham, who wrote that "the British people, left free to do so, would almost certainly have chosen to spend more on health services themselves than governments have chosen to spend on their behalf."[7] The same may be true of the single-payer systems in other countries.

To see why this is true, let us first imagine a situation in which a politician is trying to win over a single voter. To keep the example simple, suppose the politician has access to ten dollars to spend on the voter's behalf. To maximize his chance of winning, the politician should spend the ten dollars precisely as the voter wants it spent. If the voter's choice is five dollars on medical care, three dollars on a retirement pension and two dollars on a rent subsidy, that should also be the choice of the vote-maximizing politician. If the politician does not choose to spend the ten dollars in this way, he risks losing this voter to a clever opponent.

Now it might seem that if the voter wants five dollars spent on medical care, we can conclude that he would have spent the five dollars on medical care himself if he were spending ten dollars of his own money. But this is not quite true. State-provided medical care has one feature that is generally missing from private medical markets and other government spending programs—nonprice rationing. Nonprice rationing, as we have seen, imposes heavy costs on patients (the cost of waiting and other inconveniences), leads to deterioration in the quality of services rendered and creates various forms of waste and inefficiency.

Thus, other things being equal, five dollars of spending on government health care will be less valuable to the average voter than five dollars of spending in a private medical marketplace. It also means that, under socialized medicine, spending for health care will be less attractive to voters relative to spending programs that do not involve nonprice rationing.

Public choice theory, then, predicts that the average voter will desire less spending on health care, relative to other goods and services, when health care is rationed by nonmarket devices. Moreover, the greater the rationing problems, the less attractive health care spending will be. So we would expect even less spending on health care in a completely "free" service like the NHS than in a health service that charged user fees.

In the real world, politicians can rarely tailor their spending to the desires of a specific voter. Generally, they must allocate spending among programs that affect thousands of voters. New spending for a hospital, for example, provides benefits for every one in the surrounding community. And no matter what level of spending is chosen, some voters will prefer more and others less. Often, the vote-maximizing level of spending will be the level of spending preferred by the average voter.

INEQUALITIES IN HEALTH CARE

Decisions on where to spend health dollars are inherently political. A major argument in favor of national health insurance is that private medical care allows geographical inequalities in levels of provision. Yet, as we have seen, levels of provision among the geographical areas of Britain, Canada and New Zealand today may be as unequal as they would have been in the absence of national health insurance.

In theory, creating regional equality is a relatively simple task. All governments have to do is spend more in areas that are relatively deprived and less in areas that are relatively well endowed. But most governments have not done this. Why? Public choice theory supplies a possible answer.

Policy makers must make two choices about spending in a particular area or region. First, they must decide how many total dollars are to be spent there. Second, they must decide how to allocate those dollars. In a democracy, there is no particular reason why per capita spending will be the same in all areas.

Per capita spending may differ across voting districts for numerous reasons. Voter turnout may be higher in some districts than in others, which suggests that those districts are willing to "pay" more (in terms of votes) for political largesse. Voters in some districts may be more aware of, and more sensitive to, changes in per capita spending than voters in other districts.

Given that a certain amount of money is going to be spent in a certain area or region, competition for votes dictates that the money be allocated in accordance with the preference of the voters in that area or region. To return to the hypothetical example in the previous section, let us suppose that ten dollars is going to be spent in the region of Merseyside, England. If a majority of residents want two dollars spent on health services and eight dollars spent on other programs, political competition will tend to produce that result. Yet, if the residents of some other city want eight dollars spent on health services and two dollars spent on other programs, political competition will also tend to produce that result.

Prior to the establishment of national health insurance, in most developed countries geographical inequalities reflected community preferences. In general, the citizens of wealthier and more densely populated areas chose to spend a larger fraction of their income on medical care. There is no reason to suppose that their preferences were radically altered by national health insurance, and thus no reason to suppose that in allocating public spending, vote-maximizing politicians are doing anything other than responding to voter preferences.

SPENDING PRIORITIES: CARING VERSUS CURING

The British NHS's emphasis on "caring" rather than "curing" marks a radical difference between British and American health care.

There can be no doubt that Britain's choices are the result of conscious political decisions. American economist Mary-Ann Rozbicki asked a number of British health planners the following question: "If you suddenly enjoyed a sharp increase in available resources, how would you allocate it?" The response was invariably the same. They would put the additional resources into services for the aged, the chronically ill and the mentally handicapped.[8] Commenting on this response, Rozbicki writes,[9]

> It is difficult for an American observer to comprehend that view. He has been impressed by the support services already afforded the nonacute patient (and the well consumer)—the doctor, nurse and social worker attendance at homes, clinics and hospitals for the purpose of improving the comfort and well-being of the recipients involved. He has also been impressed (and sometimes shocked) by the relative lack of capability to diagnose, cure and/or treat life-threatening conditions. The U.S. patient, while having forgone the home ministrations of the family doctor and learned to endure the antiseptic quality of the hospital, also

confidently expects immediate delivery of all that medical science has to offer
if life or health is under immediate threat.

What political pressures lead decision makers to prefer caring over curing?
Rozbicki believes it is a matter of numbers: numbers of votes. Money spent on
caring affects far more people than money spent on curing. Rozbicki writes,[10]

> In weighing the choice between a more comfortable life for the millions of aged or
> early detection and treatment of the far fewer victims of dread diseases, [the British
> health authorities] have favored the former. In choosing between a fully equipped
> hospital therapy and rehabilitation center or nuclear medicine technology, they
> have favored the former. *The sheer numbers involved on each side of the equation
> would tend to dictate these choices by government officials in a democratic society.*

In the United States, almost three-quarters of health expenditure is consumed by only 10 percent of the population. As much as 41 percent of health
expenditure is consumed by the 2 percent of the population that is most in
need of care (see figure 21.1). But when health care is allocated through the

FIGURE 21-1

U.S. Distribution of Medical Costs among the Population

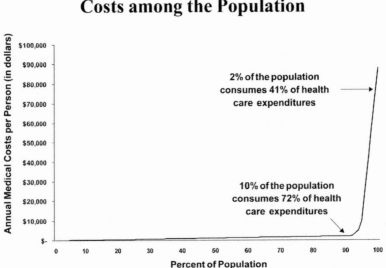

Source: Donald W. Light, "Sociological Perspectives on Competition in Health
Care," *Journal of Health Politics, Policy and Law*, October 2000.

political system, politicians cannot afford to spend 40 percent of the budget on 2 percent of the voters—people who may be too sick to get to the polls and vote in any event.

This explanation is persuasive, as far as it goes. But it is not complete. It is true that the number of potential beneficiaries of home visits far exceeds those of radiation therapy. But all Britons are potentially ill. So all have an interest in acute care, even if they do not currently need it. To understand these priorities, we must understand why the average citizen would approve of them.

Like the citizens of other countries, most Britons are relatively uninformed about the latest medical technology. This ignorance, moreover, is quite "rational." Information is costly. The rational person has an incentive to expand his knowledge about any subject only to the point at which the cost of an additional bit of information is equal to its benefit. This is the economic explanation for the commonly observed fact that the average person does not become an expert in medical science.

In Britain, however, the average citizen has much less incentive to become knowledgeable about medicine than his or her counterpart in the United States. Precisely because the U.S. medical market is largely private, a better-informed person can become a better consumer.

But under the NHS, medical services are not "purchased." Suppose a British citizen invests time and money to learn more about medical matters and discovers that the NHS is not offering the kinds of services it should. This knowledge is of almost no value unless the citizen can inform millions of other voters, persuade them to "throw the rascals out" and achieve a change of policy. Such a campaign would be enormously expensive, costing the citizen far more than he could expect to recover from any potential personal benefit.

Undoubtedly part of the reason Europeans, Canadians and citizens of many OECD countries are tolerant of single-payer health insurance systems has to do with a simple fact. Most of them are not sick. At the point of service, national health insurance makes care virtually free. The politics of medicine dictates that much of the expenditure takes place where it is consumed by the bulk of the population. The flaws of single-payer health insurance systems are most apparent where expensive intervention is needed by the few who are very ill.

Socialized medicine affects the level of knowledge that patients have in yet another way. In a free market for medical care, suppliers of medical services have an incentive to inform potential customers about new developments. Such information increases the demand for new services and, thus, promises to enhance the income of those who supply them. In the NHS, the suppliers have no such incentives. Doctors, nurses and hospital administrators increase their income chiefly by persuading the government to pay them more. They increase their comfort, leisure time and other forms of satisfaction by encouraging patients to demand not more, but less.

Public choice theory, then, would predict that under a socialized medical system, people will acquire less knowledge about medical care than they would have acquired in a private system. The evidence confirms this prediction. More than two decades ago, Rozbicki wrote that "the British populace appears much less sophisticated in its medical demands than the American populace."[11] Through the years other commentators have made the same observation and the generalization still appears to be true.

The comparative ignorance about medical science that prevails among British voters has a profound impact on NHS policies. Other things equal, people will always place a higher value on those services with which they are familiar and on benefits about which they are certain. The known is preferred to the unknown and certainty to uncertainty. The average British voter is familiar with and fairly certain about the personal value of the nonacute services provided by the NHS. He or she is probably unfamiliar with and uncertain about the personal value of advanced services for acute ailments.

Another reason why voters will tend to prefer caring to curing services stems from a characteristic of nonprice rationing. All of the services of the NHS require rationing. But in some sectors, the rationing problems are far greater than in others because quality can sometimes be sacrificed to quantity. We have seen that, in comparison with American doctors, British GPs spend less time with each patient and presumably render fewer services. Nonetheless, this type of adjustment allows the typical patient to actually visit his or her GP within two or three days of making an appointment. The quality of treatment may be inferior to what U.S. patients receive, but patients are at least certain that they will receive *some* treatment. Presumably, given the overall rationing problem, patients prefer this type of adjustment.

Such adjustments cannot be made with most acute services. It is not feasible to sacrifice quality for quantity in, for example, CT scans, organ transplants and renal dialysis. Patients either receive full treatment or no treatment, and very few patient-pleasing adjustments can be made.

These characteristics of health care rationing have an important effect on the preferences of potential patients, even those who are knowledgeable about medicine. The existence of nonprice rationing tends to make all health care services less valuable than those services would be in a free market. But because nonacute services can be adjusted to increase the certainty of some treatment, whereas acute services generally cannot, the former tend to gain value relative to the latter. Thus, the priority given to nonacute treatment seems rational.

ADMINISTRATIVE CONTROLS

One of the most remarkable features of national health insurance is the enormous amount of decision-making power left in the hands of doctors. By and large, the medical communities in Britain, Canada and New Zealand have escaped the disciplines of both the free market and government regulation. In the view of Michael Cooper,[12] Anthony Culyer[13] and many other British health economists, this discretion is the principal reason for many of the gross inefficiencies found in the British NHS.

In addition to the power of GPs and consultants, other producer interest groups have gained power and influence. Within the NHS, these include hospital administrators, junior doctors and nonmedical hospital staff. The complaint made again and again is that the NHS is primarily organized and administered to benefit such special interest groups rather than patients. As Dennis Lees puts it,[14]

> The British health industry exists for its own sake, in the interest of the producer groups that make it up. The welfare of patients is a random byproduct, depending on how conflicts between the groups and between them and government happen to shake down at any particular time.

Government production of goods and services always tends to be less efficient than private production. Nonetheless, the NHS could be run more efficiently. Its administrators could adopt well-defined goals and assert more control over the various sectors to ensure that the goals are pursued. They could create incentives for NHS employees to provide better, more efficient patient care.

That these things are not done is hardly surprising. More than 200 years ago, Adam Smith observed that government regulation in the marketplace inevitably seemed to benefit producer interest groups at the expense of consumers. Things have changed very little with the passage of time. Economic studies of virtually every major regulatory commission in the United States have come to the same conclusion: the welfare of producers is regularly favored over the welfare of consumers.[15] We should not expect the NHS to be different.

Are these phenomena consistent with public choice theory? At first glance it may seem that they are not. Since consumers outnumber producers, it might seem that, with democratic voting, consumers would always have the upper hand. If sheer voting power were the only factor, this might be so. But two additional factors put consumers at a disadvantage: the cost of information and the cost of political organization.

To achieve any fundamental change of policy, voters must be informed about what kinds of changes they specifically seek. They also must be organized—at least to the extent that they can communicate to politicians their willingness to withhold electoral support unless their desires are satisfied. But as we have seen, information is costly. Organizing a political coalition is also costly. And the incentives for any single individual to bear these costs are extremely weak.

Producers are in a different position. Since they are working in the industry, they already possess a great deal of information about which policies are consistent with their self-interest and which are not. Their costs of political organizing also are much lower because they are relatively few in number and share common interests. In addition, because the personal stake of each producer in regulatory issues is far greater than that of a representative consumer, each producer has a much greater personal incentive to contribute to political efforts that protect the interests of producers as a group.

Producer interest groups, then, ordinarily have enormous advantages over consumer groups in issues involving government regulation of their industry. These advantages appear to be more than sufficient to overcome their relative vulnerability in terms of sheer voting power. This insight was provided by Professor Milton Friedman forty years ago[16]:

> Each of us is a producer and also a consumer. However, we are much more specialized and devote a much larger fraction of our attention to our activity as a producer than as a consumer. We consume literally thousands if not millions of items. The result is that people in the same trade, like barbers or physicians, all have an intense interest in the specific problems of this trade and are willing to devote considerable energy to doing something about them. On the other hand, those of us who use barbers at all get barbered infrequently and spend only a minor fraction of our income in barber shops. Our interest is casual. Hardly any of us are willing to devote much time going to the legislature in order to testify against the inequity of restricting the practice of barbering. The same point holds for tariffs. The groups that think they have a special interest in particular tariffs are concentrated groups to whom the issue makes a great deal of difference. The public interest is widely dispersed. In consequence, in the absence of any general arrangements to offset the pressure of special interests, producer groups will invariably have a much stronger influence on legislative action and the powers that be than will the diverse, widely spread consumer interest.

Public choice theory, then, predicts that administrative inefficiencies caused by producer interest groups within health care bureaucracies will continue to be a permanent feature of socialized medicine. There is no reason to believe that this defect can be "reformed" away.

WHY THE NHS CONTINUES TO EXIST

In 1978, an article appeared in *Medical Economics* with the heading, "If Britain's Health Care Is So Bad, Why Do Patients Like It?"[17] That British patients do like the NHS had been confirmed repeatedly by public opinion polls, although its popularity has been declining.[18] And although the popularity of the Canadian health system has also been declining in Canada, Canadians show little interest in moving to a U.S.-type health care system.[19]

The principle of national health insurance is accepted in other countries for three reasons. First, the wealthy, powerful and sophisticated—those most skilled at articulating their complaints—find ways to maneuver to the front of the rationing lines. In this sense, national health insurance "works" in other countries because those who could change the system are best served by it. If a member of the British Parliament, the CEO of a large British company or the head of a major British trade union had no greater access to renal dialysis than any other British citizen, the British NHS would not last a week.

Second, those pushed to the end of the waiting lines are generally unaware of medical technologies they are being denied, at least in comparison to American patients. And, as we have seen, doctors and health authorities have little incentive to increase their level of awareness. As a result, patients in other countries frequently do not know what they are not getting.

Third, patients pushed to the rear of the waiting lines in other countries are often not very insistent about getting their needs met. A number of comparisons of British and American patients through the years have concluded that British patients are more docile.[20] Conditioned for decades by a culture of rationing, British patients put up with inadequacies that most Americans would not tolerate.

Comparing British and American patients, one doctor wrote that British patients "have fewer expectations" and are "more ready to cooperate unhesitatingly with the authoritarian figure of the doctor or nurse."[21] An American economist noted with surprise that British hospital patients, "far from complaining about specialists' inattention, a lack of laboratory tests or the ineffectiveness of medical treatment, more often than not display an attitude of gratefulness for whatever is done."[22] Another doctor summarized the difference in British and American attitudes this way[23]:

> The British people—whether as a result of different life philosophy or generally lower level of affluence—have a much lower level of expectation from medical intervention in general. In fact they verge on the stoical as compared with the

American patient, and, of course, this fact makes them, purely from a physician's point of view, the most pleasant patients. The resulting service has evolved over the years into a service that would in my opinion be all but totally unacceptable to any American not depending on welfare for medical services.

In general, the British public has little idea of how much they are paying for health care. Since the NHS is financed through hidden taxes, the perception that it costs little is widespread. Just how the perception of getting something for nothing affects British attitudes toward what most Americans would regard as intolerable defects in the health service was vividly illustrated by the experience of an American congressman on a trip with a group to examine the NHS first hand. He met a young woman with substantial facial scars received in an accident. Although the woman wanted plastic surgery for her face, she said, "I've been waiting eight years for treatment, but they tell me I'm going to be able to have surgery within a year." Yet when the congressman asked her what she thought of the NHS, her reply was, "Oh, it's a wonderful system we have in Britain. You know, our medical care is all free."[24]

It might seem that an enterprising politician or political party could win a British election by offering the British public a better deal. Why not tell voters what the NHS really costs them, then offer to return their tax dollars so they could purchase private health insurance and health services?

The average British voter would undoubtedly be better off as a result, but that doesn't mean that most would approve of the plan. For one thing, even if voters knew what the NHS really costs, they might not be convinced that the private marketplace could offer a better deal. For years, British politicians have told voters that the NHS is the "envy of the world," and the public has been deluged with stories in the socialist press indicating that only the rich get good medical care in the United States.[25]

For another thing, defenders of the NHS—including trade unions, thousands of NHS employees and many British doctors—would play on existing fears and suspicions. Surprising as it may seem, the sagging morale and continual frustrations of NHS doctors have not produced enormous numbers of converts to free enterprise medicine. Perhaps many prefer the "protection" of a government bureaucracy to the rigors of free market competition. Whatever the reason, most of Britain's medical profession supports the idea of socialized medicine.[26] They not only support it, they also resisted proposals to open it to minimal competition by prime ministers Margaret Thatcher and John Major and more recently by Tony Blair.

In almost every country with single-payer health insurance systems, disinterested, knowledgeable observers agree on the need for substantial reform. As noted, even Sweden is searching for ways to introduce the disciplines of the competitive marketplace into its public system.

There have been successful attempts to privatize public health care programs (e.g., in Singapore and Chile), and among less-developed countries there will probably be more. But among developed countries, most serious attempts at fundamental reform have been blocked by the politics of medicine. Reforms in public sector health care are likely to come about as people seek private sector alternatives rather than through changes at the ballot box.

NOTES

1. The two seminal works on public choice theory are Anthony Downs, *An Economic Theory of Democracy* (New York: Harper Row, 1957); and James Buchanan and Gordon Tullock, *The Calculus of Consent* (Ann Arbor, Mich.: University of Michigan Press, 1962). For a different approach to the theory, especially as it applies to government regulation, see George Stigler, *The Citizen and The State: Essays on Regulation* (Chicago: University of Chicago Press, 1975). See also John C. Goodman and Philip K. Porter, "Theory of Competitive Regulatory Equilibrium," *Public Choice* 59 (1988): 51–66; Gary S. Becker, "A Theory of Competition among Pressure Groups for Political Influence," *Quarterly Journal of Economics* 48, no. 3 (1983): 371–400.

2. The winning platform is not the written platform of parties (documents which tend to be ignored by voters), but the programs and policies candidates promise to implement.

3. Enoch Powell, *Medicine and Politics, 1975 and After* (New York: Pitman, 1976), 5.

4. Powell, *Medicine and Politics,* 67.

5. Goodman, *National Health Care in Great Britain: Lessons for the U.S. A.*, ch. 10.

6. Dennis Lees, "An Economist Considers Other Alternatives," in *Financing Medical Care: An Appraisal of Foreign Programs*, Helmut Schoeck, ed. (Caldwell, Idaho: Caxton Printers, 1963), 80.

7. Dennis Lees, "Economics and Non-economics of Health Services," *Three Banks Review,* no. 110 (June 1976), 9.

8. Mary-Ann Rozbicki, "Rationing British Health Care: The Cost/Benefit Approach," Executive Seminar in National and International Affairs, U.S. Department of State, April, 1978, 17.

9. Rozbicki, "Rationing British Health Care."

10. Rozbicki, "Rationing British Health Care," 18 (emphasis added).

11. Rozbicki, "Rationing British Health Care," 17.

12. Michael Cooper, *Rationing Health Care* (London: Croom Helm, 1975), 73.

13. Anthony Culyer, "Health: The Social Cost of Doctors' Discretion," *New Society* (February 27, 1975).

14. Lees, "Economics and Non-economics of Health Services," 12.

15. See Paul W. MacAvoy, ed., *Crisis of the Regulatory Commissions* (New York: Norton, 1970).

16. Milton Friedman, *Capitalism and Freedom* (Chicago: University of Chicago Press, 1962), 143.

17. John J. Fisher, "If Britain's Health Care Is So Bad, Why Do Patients Like It?" *Medical Economics* (August 21, 1978).

18. In a poll, the portion of people who were "fairly dissatisfied" or "very dissatisfied" rose to 28 percent in 1998. People reporting they were "very satisfied" fell to 13 percent, while the portion who were "fairly satisfied fell to 45 percent. Fully 90 percent of those surveyed thought the NHS needs improvement. See Annabel Ferriman, "Public's Satisfaction with the NHS Declines," *British Medical Journal* 321, no. 7275 (December 16, 2000), 1488.

19. Between 1987 and 1997, the proportion of Canadians who were satisfied with their health care system dropped from 56 percent to 20 percent. Commonwealth Fund 1998 International Health Policy Survey, cited in Karen Donelan et al., "The Cost of Health System Change: Public Discontent in Five Nations," *Health Affairs* 18, no. 3 (May/June 1999), 206–16, Exhibit 6.

20. For a comparison of how patient attitudes and treatments vary by culture, see Lynn Payer, *Medicine and Culture* (New York: Henry Holt, 1996).

21. Derek Robinson, "Primary Medical Practice in the United Kingdom and the United States," *New England Journal of Medicine* 297, no. 4 (July 28, 1977): 189.

22. Rozbicki, "Rationing British Health Care," 18.

23. Quoted in Harry Swartz, "The Infirmity of British Medicine," in *The Future That Doesn't Work: Social Democracy's Failures in Britain*, Emmett Tyrrell Jr., ed. (New York: Doubleday, 1977), 31.

24. Quoted by Lew Rockwell in *World Research INC*, March 1979, 5.

25. Quoted by Lew Rockwell in *World Research INC*, March 1979, 6.

26. John Walsh, "Britain's National Health Service: the Doctors' Dilemmas," *Science* 201 (July 28, 1979), 329.

Chapter Twenty-two

Is Managed Competition the Answer?[1]

Most of the problems of single-payer health care insurance are well known to policy makers and government officials and even to many ordinary citizens in countries with national health insurance. Many of the obstacles posed by the politics of medicine also are well known.

As a result, throughout the 1990s there was growing interest—particularly in Europe—in a new type of system, one in which health care resources would be allocated by competition in the marketplace rather than by politicians. Such a system would not be a free market in the ordinary sense of that term; rather it would be a market in which the rules of competition were set and managed by government. So long as the competitors played by the rules, market forces rather than political forces would determine who got health care and how much. Such a system is called managed competition. And to obtain a model of it, Europeans turned, of all places, to the United States.[2]

Employees, for example, of the federal government make an annual choice among a dozen or more competing health plans.[3] A similar choice system is in place for employees of many state and local governments.[4] Many private employers also give employees a choice of health plans, and where these plans are independent organizations they effectively compete against each other to enroll members.[5]

The competition that exists in these programs, again, is not the same as one would find in a free market. It takes place under artificial rules managed by the employer or some other sponsoring organization. During its first term, the Clinton administration proposed such managed competition nationwide. Its adherents, including Stanford professor Alain Enthoven, still think this is the answer to the nation's health care woes.[6]

MANAGED COMPETITION

Under the health insurance options described above, health plans do indeed compete. But because the way they compete is artificially constrained, the product they sell is different from garden-variety health insurance. For example, each health plan is required to charge the same premium to every applicant (community rating) or to every applicant of the same age and sex (modified community rating) and to accept all applicants regardless of health conditions (guaranteed issue). In the federal employees program, for example, an eighty-year-old retiree pays the same premium to join a health plan as a twenty-year-old employee.[7] As a result, insurers are precluded from competing on their ability to price and manage risk. Instead, they must compete on their ability to provide health care and manage its cost. Such competition is not really competition among firms in the business of insurance; instead, it is competition in the delivery of health care.

The artificial market changes the nature of the product not only for the sellers, but also for the buyers. Buyers are not purchasing protection against the loss of their assets when they select one of these health plans. The system as a whole provides protection against the loss of assets due to an expensive illness. What customers are selecting is the right to particular health care services, such as access to one doctor network rather than another. This is comparable to choosing an auto insurer so you can have your car repaired at a particular auto repair shop or choosing a casualty insurer so you can get hail damage repair from a particular roofer.

The benefits of competition are well known to economists and to many noneconomists. These benefits flow principally from the fact that sellers find it in their self-interest to compete for the trade of potential customers. To do so, they make buyer-pleasing adjustments in their competitive strategies. However, none of the valuable benefits of competition can be expected to emerge if sellers find it in their self-interest not to sell to some buyers and if they compete with each other to avoid such customers. Yet, these are the perverse incentives that managed competition creates.

People who know before they select an insurer that they need expensive medical treatment will use this knowledge to select a health plan. And since insurers understand this, they can structure their products so as to discourage the most expensive customers. Let's look at some ways this might happen.

HOW PERVERSE INCENTIVES
AFFECT THE BEHAVIOR OF BUYERS

Imagine a system in which health plans offer networks of doctors and hospitals in return for fixed premiums. People who are seriously ill and need specific, expensive medical treatment will select in a very different way from other people. Take a heart patient in need of cardiovascular surgery. The individual has a self-interest in finding the best cardiologist and the best heart clinic. Armed with this knowledge, the patient will try to learn which health plan employs the cardiologist or has a contract with the clinic. The premium matters little, since the value to the patient of receiving the best cardiovascular care will far exceed any premium payment.

The incentives facing healthy people are different. Since their probability of needing any particular service in the near future is small, they are unlikely to spend much time investigating particular doctors and clinics. To the degree that they do investigate, they are likely to inquire only about the primary care services they are likely to receive. If the need for heart surgery arises, odds are that patients will be able to switch insurers before the surgery is performed.

Thus, the people who carefully compare the acute care services offered by competing health plans are likely to be the people who intend to use them. These are the very people health plans want to avoid. By contrast, those who choose a plan based on the quality and accessibility of nonacute services are more likely to be healthy.

HOW PERVERSE INCENTIVES
AFFECT THE BEHAVIOR OF SELLERS

To see how managed competition affects the incentives of insurers, imagine two competing HMOs. In the first, enrollees can see a primary care physician at any time, but there are cumbersome screening mechanisms and waiting periods for kidney dialysis, heart surgery and other expensive procedures. In the second, dialysis and heart surgery are available when needed, but primary care facilities are limited. Given a choice, most of us would enroll in the first HMO if we were healthy and switch to the second if afflicted with heart disease or kidney failure. But if everyone acted in this way, the second HMO would attract only expensive-to-treat patients. To cover its costs, it would have to charge a premium many times higher than the first HMO. The premium would have to be approximately equal to the cost of heart surgery or a kidney transplant. But in that case, most people could not afford the premium. Those who could afford it might be better off to simply buy their medical care directly. In any event, the HMO would face financial ruin.[8]

It might seem that the second HMO could compete successfully by offering more primary care services. But to be truly competitive, it would have to change its strategy completely. The easiest way to keep costs down is to enroll only the healthy. And the easiest way to do that is not to have the doctors and facilities sick people want. As Alain Enthoven has noted (disapprovingly), "A good way to avoid enrolling diabetics is to have no endocrinologists on staff. . . . A good way to avoid cancer patients is to have a poor oncology department."[9]

To attract healthy enrollees, a health plan might offer inexpensive vaccinations, cancer screening and health club membership. The plan also might offer services at more convenient times and locations, free parking and other amenities. Of course, these services might be attractive to all potential applicants, but they are more likely to be decisive for healthy people. Health plans also can target the healthy through the design of their advertisements and in selecting a location to make a pitch to desirable prospects.

A survey by the Kaiser Family Foundation discovered how HMOs were competing for seniors on Medicare. The HMO ads in print and on television showed seniors snorkeling, biking and swimming, but did not feature the sick or disabled. In addition, nearly one-third of HMO marketing seminars were held at sites that were not wheelchair accessible.[10] The following are just a few other examples uncovered by the *Washington Post*[11]:

- When a Minnesota network began offering direct access to an obstetrician while rivals required referrals from a gatekeeper, it attracted disproportionate numbers of pregnant women, lost millions of dollars and soon ended the practice.
- When Aetna U.S. Healthcare offered unusually generous coverage for in vitro fertilization, people with fertility problems flocked to the HMO and Aetna had to end the practice.
- In another case, a California health plan severed its relationship with a university hospital known for practicing high-tech medicine and tackling complicated cases.
- Other HMOs avoid contracting with doctors' groups known for expertise with high-risk patients.

The term *medlining* is sometimes used to describe the practice of avoiding the sick. It's health care's version of redlining, the banking and insurance practice of avoiding deteriorating neighborhoods. The other side of the coin, of course, is attracting the healthy. In addition to health club memberships, health plans also have offered dental benefits and vision care. The theory is that anyone who will switch health plans to get a free pair of eyeglasses cannot be very sick.[12]

THE RESULTS OF COMPETITION

In figure 22.1, patients are arrayed along the horizontal axis from most to least costly (left to right). The cost-of-care line shows what would be spent on each patient given current standards of medical practice. This line is highly skewed, reflecting the fact that in a typical pool about 2 percent of the group spends more than 40 percent of the health care dollars, 10 percent spends almost three-quarters and the majority have very small expenses. The premium is based on the average cost of care for all patients under community rating. It is the premium that must be charged all plan members if the plan is to cover its costs.[13] The figure also illustrates how healthy people subsidize sick people, since most members have costs well below the premium they pay and a few have costs well above it. Clearly, this is what many proponents of managed competition believe equilibrium would look like for each health plan under their scheme. But simple analysis shows that the diagram in figure 22.1 cannot be in equilibrium and that it must give way to something else.

Roughly speaking, an equilibrium exists if no health plan can adjust to become more profitable.[14] However, the plan represented in figure 22.1 can easily become more profitable if it can lower the cost of caring for its sicker members. As long as these members stay in the plan, it will have the same premium income and lower costs. If sicker members shift to another plan, this is even better from the plan's point of view—since the sick are unprofitable by definition. On the other hand, healthier customers are being overcharged, since the cost of care they are receiving is below the premium they are paying. This means that other health plans can lure away these customers by providing higher benefits for the same premium. Thus, in order to retain prof-

FIGURE 22-1

Disequilibrium for a Health Plan Under Managed Competition

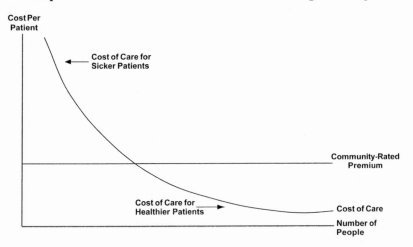

FIGURE 22-2

Competitive Pressures under Managed Competition

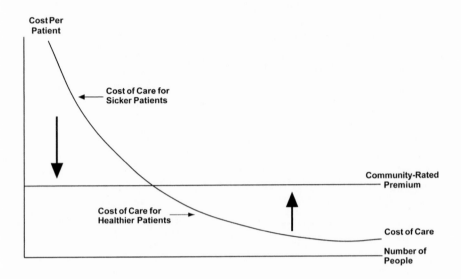

itable customers and attract even more, the health plan represented in figure 22.1 should increase the amount it spends on healthy members.

In free markets, competition tends to cause the price to change until it equals average cost. The same tendencies exist under artificial competition. Yet, because community-rated premiums are constrained to be the same for all members, competition will cause cost to change until it equals price. If premiums could rise for "unprofitable" members, health plans would compete them up to the level of the cost of those people's care. But if the premiums are artificially constrained, the plans will compete the cost of care down to the level of the artificial premium.[15] The reverse pressures exist for "profitable" members. If the artificial premiums cannot be competed down to the level of average cost, the tendency will be to compete cost up to the level of the artificial premium.

These conclusions follow from well-known principles of the economics of regulation. In the United States, we have had decades of experience with regulated markets. Under regulations imposed by the Civil Aeronautics Board (CAB) for most of the post–World War II period, the federal government established minimum air fares higher than would have prevailed in a free market. Unable to compete on price, the airlines competed by offering more frequent flights, more convenient departures, more spacious seating and other in-flight amenities. The CAB's price regulation potentially allowed the airlines to earn supra-normal profits, but those profits were competed away on passenger-pleasing adjustments.[16]

The reverse tendency emerges when prices are kept artificially low. Under rent control laws, landlords are prohibited from raising their rents to the level of average cost. Since rents cannot rise, landlords tend to allow housing quality to deteriorate until housing costs equal the government-controlled rent.[17]

Consider this result in terms of a basic principle taught in all introductory economics courses: when firms are maximizing profits, marginal revenue must equal marginal cost. Under artificial competition, marginal revenue (the amount of premium each additional enrollee brings to a plan) must be the same for every enrollee. Thus, if health plans are maximizing profits, marginal cost (the amount the plan spends on the health care of each additional enrollee) also must be the same for every enrollee.

Health plans, therefore, face competitive pressures to adjust the delivery of health care until the cost-of-care line coincides with the (community-rated) premium line (see figure 22.2). This means that health plans have a strong financial self-interest in underproviding services to the sick and overproviding services to the healthy. Left unchecked, the end result of this process is a condition under which each person receives health services whose cost is exactly equal to the premium he or she pays.

THE EFFECT OF LIMITED OPEN SEASONS

The analysis presented here assumes that patients make choices among insurers based solely on the value of medical services those patients consume. This assumption would be justified to the degree that patients can easily shift back and forth among insurers as their health needs change. However, the federal employee program and most other managed competition programs allow plan changes only during "open season" once a year.[18]

To the degree that people's choices are constrained by limited open seasons, they must consider the insurance value of the plan they select as well as its direct consumption value. Consider an expectant mother choosing among competing health plans. She expects to need well-baby delivery services. However, she might experience complications in pregnancy or childbirth, or her child might be premature and require sophisticated medical treatment. In those cases, the woman would benefit from highly skilled medical personnel. Thus, in selecting a plan she will be interested in purchasing real insurance as well as specific medical services.

For such potential problems as heart disease, cancer and AIDS, it seems unlikely that people will willingly pay much to insure for expensive treatment while they are healthy—if they can switch insurers at least every twelve months. The tendency will be to select a plan that is strong on preventive and diagnostic services, secure in the knowledge that one can rather quickly switch to a plan that is best at treating a particular disease.

Therefore, periodic open seasons cause us to modify our prediction in recognition of an insurance component to people's choices. Yet, even with this modification we are left with the prediction that artificial competition will ultimately result in a radical deterioration in the quality of care sick people receive.

THE EFFECT OF RISK ADJUSTMENT

Proponents of managed competition are keenly aware of the perverse incentives faced by health plans. To thwart these incentives many favor risk adjustment programs that take income away from plans that attract healthier people and give it to plans that attract sicker people.

Many methods of risk adjustment have been suggested. None of them work very well. It might seem that the logical way to start constructing a risk adjustment mechanism would be to tax or subsidize health plans based on the health of people at the time they joined a plan. Thus, sicker people would have a subsidy added to their premium payments and healthier people would have a tax deducted from theirs. Although enrollees would pay the same community-rated premium, health plans would receive a risk adjusted premium. In theory, this would make the health plans indifferent between potential enrollees.

The problem with this approach is that it does not work very well. Health economist Joseph Newhouse notes that in the RAND Health Insurance Experiment, 1 percent of the patients accounted for 28 percent of the total costs, but most of the high-cost patients could not have been identified in advance. In fact, Newhouse found that only 15 percent of the variation in health care costs among individuals could be predicted in advance, even when researchers had full knowledge of the patients' demographic characteristics.[19] More recently, Newhouse and his colleagues have concluded that as much as 25 percent of the variation in health expenditures for individuals can be predicted by such observable factors as health status and prior health expenditure.[20] That leaves 75 percent unexplained.

Some health economists argue that it doesn't matter whether a risk adjustment mechanism is perfect. As long as the adjuster predicts as well as the health plans themselves, the adjuster can remove any financial incentives a plan has to prefer or avoid a person at the time of enrollment. Yet, this does not solve the problem for two reasons. First, after an initial enrollment, everyone will be a member of a health plan. Therefore, at least one plan can probably predict that member's future health costs better than an impersonal risk adjuster that relies only on statistical data. Second, the perverse incentives of health plans do not end at the point of enrollment. To the contrary, health plans do not have to be able to predict which enrollees will get heart attacks in order to know that it doesn't pay to invest too much in cardiology. The incentive to underprovide to the sick is ongoing, 365 days a year.

If adjustments cannot solve the problem based on prior knowledge of patients, the only alternative is to base them on knowledge of the experiences of patients after they enroll.[21] But if we do that, how much should the plan be paid? Consider again the cost-of-care line in figure 22.2. If the net amount insurers received for each applicant were based on this line rather than on the artificial premium line, insurers would have no reason to overprovide or underprovide care to any enrollee. The problem is that we never get to observe what the efficient cost-of-care line looks like. All an outside observer can see is the actual amount spent. And if we reimbursed health plans for actual expenditures, health plans would have no incentive to provide efficient care. Indeed, the practice of paying providers based on their costs was what led to so much health care inefficiency before the managed care revolution. Whatever the defects of managed care, a return to cost-plus finance is not the answer.[22]

An alternative to paying health plans based on actual costs is to pay fixed fees determined by the patient's diagnosis. This is the way Medicare reimburses hospitals, and it has produced some efficiencies. The reason is that hospitals get to keep the diagnosis-related payment, regardless of actual costs. So the lower their actual costs, the higher their profit or the lower their losses. The disadvantage of this approach is that fixed payment is almost always based on expected average cost for patients with a particular condition. By definition, the sum fails to cover the treatment costs of the sickest patients. The more competitive the market, the greater the pressure is to underprovide to the patients whose cost of care is above average.[23]

Regardless of how risk adjustment is carried out, it can at best ameliorate the problem of quality. It cannot solve it. Even if premiums vary with changes in expected costs, the underlying economics are the same. Health plans here have an incentive to adjust the quality of care they deliver until they are spending an amount on each enrollee equal to that enrollee's risk-adjusted premium.

OTHER BARRIERS TO QUALITY DETERIORATION

Just because health plans have an economic incentive to let treatment costs
fall until they are no greater than the premium payments made on behalf of
the sickest patients does not mean they will do so. Fear of tort liability lawsuits is one obstacle to quality deterioration. Doctors' fear of censure or loss
of a license to practice is another. But these obstacles are somewhat crude in-
struments for combating incentives that affect every decision providers make.

MANAGED COMPETITION VERSUS
SINGLE-PAYER NATIONAL HEALTH INSURANCE

The most serious defect of national health insurance is the tendency to overprovide to the healthy and underprovide to the sick. This, we have seen, occurs because of the pressures inherent in allocating health care resources
through the political system. Politicians cannot afford to spend most of the
health care budget on the small number who need expensive care. Democratic
politics forces them to take from the sick and give to the healthy instead.

However, managed competition, whatever efficiencies it produces, cannot
solve this problem. In fact it may make the problem worse. Whereas national
health insurance overprovides to the healthy and underprovides to the sick for
political reasons, managed competition leads to a similar result because of
perverse economic incentives.

MANAGED COMPETITION
VERSUS MARKET-DRIVEN HEALTH CARE

One of the ironies of health policy is that some of the strongest critics of national health insurance are also some of the strongest advocates of managed
competition; Alain Enthoven is one example. Yet, the closer we come to the
ideal world of managed competition, the more likely we are to experience
outcomes similar to those of socialized medicine. Moreover, this conclusion
is not tied to the design of any particular employer plan. There is a sense in
which our entire employer-based system functions as a loose system of managed competition.

Ordinarily, we think of the labor market as being literally a market for labor, with health insurance tacked on as a fringe benefit. But imagine for a mo-
ment that it were the other way around. Imagine that employers offered health
plans with the provision that you must take a job in order to enroll. Farfetched

as the latter scenario may seem, it is precisely the way thousands of people view the job market. These are people with high health costs or people with a dependent family member whose health costs are high. For this group of potential employees, employers offer competitive health plans—all heavily subsidized and all community rated. The employees switch plans by switching jobs; and because their health costs are so high, the kind of work they agree to do becomes a secondary concern. In fact, they are willing to take jobs for which they are overqualified (a college graduate working in a mailroom, for example) just to access a benefit-rich health care plan.

To large employers with generous health plans, the scenario we are describing is not fanciful. These companies confront similar problems everyday. Indeed, a major reason why K-Mart, Wal-Mart and other large retail chain stores have cut back on their health benefits is not that they are stingy; it is that they were attracting individuals and families with very high health care costs.[24] In protecting themselves from adverse labor market selection, these companies are engaging in the exact behavior predicted by the economic theory of managed competition.

The United States is in danger of evolving a system that underprovides to the sick, not because we have made a conscious decision to socialize health care, but because we have created perverse economic incentives for employers and their employees.

NOTES

1. This section is largely based on John C. Goodman and Gerald L. Musgrave, "A Primer on Managed Competition," National Center for Policy Analysis, Policy Report No. 183, April 1994.

2. See the brief discussion in the Introduction.

3. The Federal Employees Health Benefits Program (FEHBP) has four main features: (1) federal employees in most places can choose among eight to 12 competing health insurance plans, including Blue Cross and a number of HMOs; (2) the government contributes a fixed amount that can be as much as 75 percent of each employee's premium; (3) the extra cost of more expensive plans must be paid by the employee with aftertax dollars; and (4) the plans are forced to community rate, charging the same premium for every enrollee. Public employee health benefit options in the state of Minnesota are similarly organized, as is the California Public Employees' Retirement System (CalPERS).

4. Bryan Dowd and Roger D. Feldman, "Employer Premium Contributions and Health Insurance Costs." in *Managed Care and Changing Health Care Markets*, Michael Morrisey, ed. (Washington, D.C.: American Enterprise Institute, 1998): 24–54.

5. James Maxwell et al., "Managed Competition in Practice: 'Value Purchasing' by Fourteen Employers," *Health Affairs* 17, no. 3 (May/June 1998): 216–27.

6. The case for managed competition was forcefully argued in Alain Enthoven, *Health Plan: The Only Practical Solution to the Soaring Cost of Medical Care* (Reading, Mass.: Addison-Wesley, 1980). For an update on Enthoven's views on the advantages and disadvantages of the FEHBP, see Enthoven, "Effective Management of Competition in the FEHBP," *Health Affairs* 8, no. 3 (Fall 1989): 33–50.

7. Congress initially exempted itself and other government employees from Medicare coverage, which meant that younger federal employees had to directly subsidize the premiums of eighty- and ninety-year-old retirees. The policy was changed for new employees in the early 1980s so that 80 to 85 percent of federal employees now have Medicare coverage—and Medicare is the payer of first resort.

8. The HMO would receive premiums only from people who were about to undergo expensive medical procedures. Thus, the average premium would have to equal the average cost of the procedures. It is precisely because most people cannot easily bear such a financial burden that health insurance is desirable in the first place.

9. Alain Enthoven, "The History and Principles of Managed Competition," *Health Affairs* (1993 Supplement), 35. On the practice of encouraging high-cost patients to "disenroll," see Jonathan E. Fielding and Thomas Rice, "Can Managed Competition Solve the Problems of Market Failure?" *Health Affairs* (1993 Supplement): 222; and Joseph Newhouse, "Is Competition the Answer?" *Journal of Health Economics* 1, no. 1 (January 1982): 109–16.

10. Reported in Natalie Hopkinson, "Study Finds Medicare HMOs Target Active Seniors but Not Disabled in Ads," *Wall Street Journal*, July 14, 1998.

11. David Hilzenrath, "Showing the Sickest Patients the Door," *Washington Post, National Weekly Edition*, February 2, 1998.

12. Hilzenrath, "Showing the Sickest."

13. Note that the premium does not have to be the same for all plans, but it must be the same for all members of a given plan.

14. More formally, an equilibrium is said to exist when no participant in the market—including all buyers and sellers—can improve his or her position by any unilateral move.

15. Other analysts have recognized this problem, noting that the tendency is one of "the free market pitfalls of managed competition" (p. 118), that "one of managed competition's greatest challenges is to safeguard quality of care without robbing the system of free-market efficiencies" (p. 110) and that "managed competition carries an inherent risk of discrimination against enrollees who incur high health care costs" (p. 120). See Alan L. Hillman, William R. Greer and Neil Goldfarb, "Safeguarding Quality in Managed Competition," *Health Affairs* (1993 Supplement): 110–22.

16. Edwin S. Dolan and John C. Goodman, "Flying the Deregulated Skies: Competition, Price Discrimination, Congestion," in *Economics of Public Policy,* 5th ed. (St. Paul: West Publishing Co., 1995): 143–59.

17. See William Tucker, *The Excluded Americans: Homelessness and Housing Policies* (Washington, D.C.: Regnery Gateway, 1990).

18. The Jackson Hole Group and other proponents of managed competition argue that open enrollment periods should be infrequent. See Michael Moore, "Risk Adjustment under Managed Competition," Jackson Hole draft discussion paper, March 1993.

19. See Joseph P. Newhouse, "Rate Adjusters for Medicare under Capitation," *Health Care Financing Review* (1986 Annual Supplement): 45–56, cited in Alain Enthoven, "The History and Principles of Managed Competition," *Health Affairs* (Supplement 1993): 24–48.

20. Joseph P. Newhouse, Melinda Beeuwkes Buntin and John D. Chapman, "Risk Adjustment and Medicare: Taking a Closer Look," *Health Affairs* 16, no. 5 (September/October 1997): 26–43.

21. See Harold S. Luft, "Compensating for Biased Selection in Health Insurance," *Milbank Quarterly* 64 (1986): 580; and Alain Enthoven, *Theory and Practice of Managed Competition in Health Care Finance* (New York: Elsevier Science Publishing Co., 1988), 86; and Newhouse, Buntin and Chapman, "Risk Adjustment and Medicare," 34–35.

22. For a discussion of the cost-plus system, see John C. Goodman and Gerald L. Musgrave, *Patient Power: Solving America's Health Care Crisis* (Washington, D.C.: Cato Institute, 1992), chs. 5–9.

23. Under the Prospective Payment System (PPS), there are 503 diagnostic-related groups (DRGs), and physicians and hospitals receive a predetermined amount from the federal government for whatever services they perform. See Goodman and Musgrave, *Patient Power*: 303–6.

24. Bernard Wysocki Jr. and Ann Zimmerman, "Wal-Mart Cost-Cutting Finds a Big Target in Health Benefits," *Wall Street Journal*, September 30, 2003.

Part Three

REFORMING THE U.S. HEALTH CARE SYSTEM

Chapter Twenty-three

Designing an Ideal
Health Care System

Among people who believe the American health care system needs serious reform, attention invariably turns to the large number of people without health insurance. An estimated 43.6 million people, or 15.2 percent of the U.S. population, were without coverage for at least part of 2002.[1] What can be done about this problem?

There are typically two types of proposals: (1) force people to buy private health insurance whether they want to or not, or force their employers to buy it for them (which amounts to the same thing)[2]; and (2) have government pay for all or most of the cost of their insurance by subsidizing private premiums or enrolling them in public insurance.

The first proposal not only involves government coercion, but also constitutes a dangerous further intrusion of government into the medical marketplace. The second proposal would require new taxes and inject billions of additional dollars into a health care system that is already the most expensive in the world.

As we shall see in the next chapter, neither reform is necessary or desirable. In fact, we can have a workable form of universal health insurance without intrusive mandates or more government spending.

THE ROLE OF GOVERNMENT

But before turning to a solution, we should consider a more basic question. Why should government be involved at all?

The Free Rider Argument

Aside from the burden of providing charity care to the poor, is there any reason for government to care whether people have health insurance? The traditional argument for government intervention is that health insurance has social benefits apart from the personal benefits to the person who chooses to insure. The reason is that people who fail to insure are likely to get health care anyway, even if they can't pay for it. And the reason for that is that the rest of the community is unwilling to allow the uninsured to go without health care, even if their lack of insurance is willful and negligent.

This set of circumstances creates opportunities for some people to be free riders on other people's generosity. In particular, free riders can choose not to pay insurance premiums and to spend the money on other consumption instead—confident that the community as a whole will provide them with care even if they cannot pay for it when they need it. In other words, being a free rider works. It works because of a tacit community agreement that no one will be allowed to go without health care. And this tacit agreement is so established that it operates as a social contract that many people substitute for a private insurance contract.

Evidence of a Free Rider Problem:
The Growing Number of Uninsured

What evidence is there that free riders are a problem? One piece of evidence is the number of uninsured. According to the Census Bureau, a larger percentage of the population was uninsured in 2002 than a decade earlier (see figure 23.1). The rise in the number of uninsured occurred throughout the 1990s, a time in which per capita income and wealth, however measured, were rising.

Although it is common to think of the uninsured as having low incomes, many families who lack insurance are solidly middle class (see figure 23.2). And the largest increase in the number of uninsured in recent years has occurred among higher-income families:

- About one in six uninsured persons lives in a family with an income between $50,000 and $75,000, and almost one in six earns more than $75,000.
- Further, between 1993 and 1999, the number of uninsured increased by 57 percent in households earning between $50,000 to $75,000 and by 114 percent among households earning $75,000 or more.
- By contrast, in households earning less than $50,000 the number of uninsured decreased approximately 2 percent.

FIGURE 23-1

Growth in the Uninsured, 1990 to 2002
(millions)

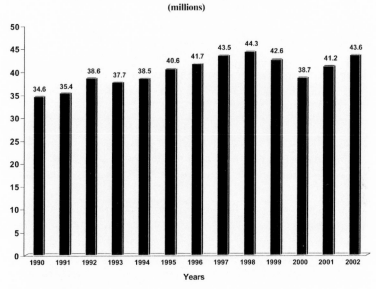

Source: U.S. Census Bureau.

FIGURE 23-2

Income Distribution of the Uninsured
(2002)

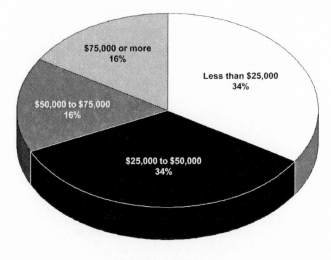

Sources: Robert J. Mills, *Current Population Reports. Health Insurance Coverage: 1999*, :60-211, U.S. Census Bureau, September 2000.

More information about middle-class families who are voluntarily uninsured emerged from a recent California survey of the uninsured with incomes
of more than 200 percent of poverty.[3]

- 40 percent owned their own homes and more than half owned a personal
  computer.
- 20 percent worked for an employer that offered health benefits, but half of
  them (10 percent of the total) declined coverage for which they were eligible.
- This group was not opposed to insurance in general, as 90 percent had purchased auto, home or life insurance in the past.
- About 43 percent felt that health insurance was not a good value for the
  money, and rising insurance premiums will only increase this number.

These results are contrary to the normal expectation of economists. Economic theory teaches that as people earn higher incomes, they should be
more willing to purchase insurance to protect their income against claims
arising from expensive medical bills. Similarly, as people become wealthier
the value of insuring against wealth depletion (say, by a catastrophic illness)
rises. So insurance should be positively correlated with income and wealth
accumulation. The fact that the number of uninsured rose while incomes
were rising and that the greatest increase in lack of insurance was among
higher-income families suggests that something else is making insurance
less attractive.

Cause of the Problem:
State Regulations That Favor Free Ridership

One cause of the problem is the proliferation of state laws that make it increasingly easy for people to obtain insurance after they get sick. Guaranteed
issue regulations (requiring insurers to take all comers, regardless of health
status) and community-rating regulations (requiring insurers to charge the
same premium to all enrollees, regardless of health status) are a free rider's
heaven. They encourage everyone to remain uninsured while healthy, confident that they can obtain insurance if they get sick.

Moreover, as healthy people respond to these incentives by electing to be
uninsured, the premium that must be charged to cover costs for those who remain in insurance pools rises. These higher premiums, in turn, encourage
even more healthy people to drop their coverage. From 1990 through 1996,
sixteen states passed aggressive regulations to increase access to health in-

surance for people with health problems. The uninsured population in these states grew eight times as much as in the states that did not do this.[4]

Other regulations that raise the cost of insurance for the healthy exacerbate this condition. Among these are laws mandating coverage for such services as acupuncture, in vitro fertilization and even marriage counseling.[5] For example, a Duke University study showed that the probability an individual will become uninsured increases with each new mandate imposed by government.[6] A study for the Health Insurance Association of America (HIAA) found that 20 percent to 25 percent of uninsured Americans lack insurance due to benefit mandates.[7]

Cause of the Problem:
Federal Regulations That Favor Free Ridership

Federal legislation has also made it increasingly easy to obtain insurance after one gets sick. HIPAA (1996) had a noble intent: guarantee that people who have been paying premiums into the private insurance system do not lose coverage simply because they change jobs. But a side effect of pursuing this desirable goal is a provision that allows any small business to obtain insurance regardless of the health status of its employees. This means that a small operation can save money by remaining uninsured until a family member gets sick. Individuals can also opt out of their employer's plan, then enroll after they get sick. They are entitled to full coverage for a preexisting condition after an eighteen-month waiting period.[8]

Cause of the Problem:
National Spending on Indigent Health Care

Another source of the problem is the amount we spend on free care for those who cannot or do not pay their own medical bills. As noted earlier in this book, public and private spending on free care is considerable. For example, a study by the State Comptroller's office found that Texas currently spends about $1,000 per year on free care for every uninsured person in the state, on the average. This implies that the value of "free" care is about $4,000 a year for a family of four.

Interestingly, $4,000 is a sum adequate to purchase private health insurance for a family in many Texas cities. Therefore, many Texas families can rely on $4,000 in free care (on the average) or they can purchase a $4,000 private insurance policy with after-tax income. Granted, the two alternatives are not exactly comparable. Families surely have more options if they

FIGURE 23-3

Health Spending on the Uninsured in Texas

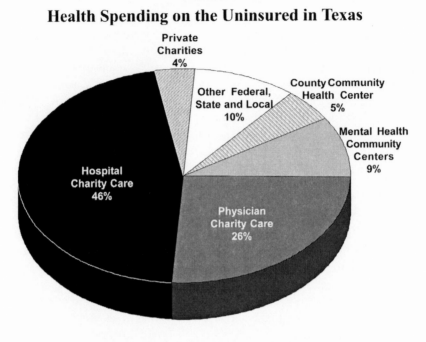

Source: Estimated Texas Health Care Spending on the Uninsured, Texas
Comptroller's Office, May 9, 2000.

have private insurance. But to many, the free care alternative appears more attractive.[9]

Consequences of Free Ridership:
An Increasingly Fragile Safety Net

As we shall see below, when people elect to become insured, say by enrolling in an employer's health plan, they receive a tax subsidy from the federal government. However, when people drop insurance coverage the federal government makes no extra contribution to any local health care safety net. As a consequence, the growth in the uninsured is straining the finances of many urban hospitals. The problem is exacerbated by less generous federal reimbursement for Medicaid and Medicare and by increasing competitiveness in the hospital sector. Traditionally, hospitals have covered losses that arise from people who can't pay for their care by overcharging those who can. But as the market becomes more competitive, these overcharges are shrinking. There is no such thing as "cost shifting" in a competitive market.

This problem is not trivial. For example, preliminary findings from one study show that safety net spending by the nation's hospitals is not keeping pace with the overall increase in per capita spending.[10] A National Academy of Sciences Institute of Medicine study found that the safety net of local clinics, hospitals and charities is "overburdened and threadbare" and "could collapse with disastrous consequences."[11]

CHARACTERISTICS OF AN IDEAL HEALTH CARE SYSTEM

Even if federal, state and local governments did not exacerbate the problem of the uninsured, some people would choose to be uninsured, giving rise to the "free rider" argument outlined above. Yet, if this is the reason why government has a legitimate interest in the health insurance decisions of individuals, then the public policies we adopt must solve the problem. As noted, the most commonly proposed solutions are to have government require people to purchase insurance and/or have taxpayers subsidize their insurance. Yet, government-imposed mandates and expensive new spending programs are neither necessary nor sufficient. The best solution limits the role of government and expands the choices open to every citizen. Here's how:

Characteristic No. 1: We Should Reward Those Who Insure and Penalize Those Who Do Not

To the advocates of mandates, we can always ask the question: What are you going to do with people who disobey the mandate? As a practical matter, no one is suggesting that we put them in jail. So we are left with imposing a financial penalty (e.g., a fine). But a system that fines people who are uninsured is a system that subsidizes those who insure—the subsidy being the absence of the fine.

Under the current system families who obtain insurance through an employer get a tax subsidy worth about $1,155, on the average.[12] Since an uninsured family with an average income doesn't get this subsidy, the uninsured family will pay about $1,155 more in taxes. So instead of describing our current system as one that subsidizes employer-provided insurance we could, with equal validity, describe it as one that penalizes the lack of employer-provided insurance.

We can describe any incentive system in one of two ways: (1) as one that grants subsidies to those who insure and withholds them from those who do not or (2) as one that taxes the uninsured and refrains from taxing the insured. Either description is valid, since a reward is simply the mirror image of a penalty.

Characteristics of an Ideal Health Care System

Characteristic No. 1: We should subsidize those who insure and
penalize those who do not.

Characteristic No. 2: The subsidy/penalty should equal the value
society places on insuring individuals, at the
margin.

Characteristic No. 3: The revealed social value of insurance is the
amount we spend on free care for the unin-
sured.

Characteristic No. 4: The tax penalties paid by the uninsured
should be used to compensate those who
provide safety net care.

Characteristic No. 5: The tax subsidies for the insured should, at
the margin, be funded by reducing spending
on free care for the uninsured.

Characteristic No. 6: Subsidies for being insured should be independent of how the insurance is purchased.

Characteristic No. 7: The optimal number of uninsured is not zero.

Characteristic No. 8: The principles of reform apply with equal
force to all citizens, regardless of income.

Characteristic No. 9: Health insurance subsidies need not add to
budgetary outlays.

Characteristic No. 10: The federal government's role should remain
strictly financial.

Characteristic No. 2: The Reward/Penalty Should Equal the Value Society Places on Insuring Individuals at the Margin

We should decide how much we care (in money terms) whether a person is insured or not and that should determine the size of the subsidy/penalty.[13] Any other policy would be indefensible and absurd. It would entail spending too much on subsidies and collecting too much in fines, or vice versa. Under an ideal system,

FIGURE 23-4

Average Tax Subsidy for Families

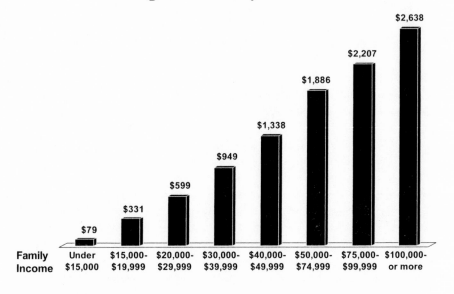

Note: Includes subsidy from the income tax exclusion, the Social Security income tax
 exclusion and the health expenses deduction.

Source: Lewin Group estimates.

- We should never pay more for (reward) good behavior than the good behavior's benefit to us, and we should never collect more from (penalize) bad behavior than its cost to us.
- Conversely, we should never pay less for good behavior than its benefit or penalize bad behavior less than its cost.

Current policy violates this principle in several ways. Although the average tax subsidy is worth about $1,155 per family, households earning more than $100,000 per year receive, on the average, $2,638 per year in subsidies. By contrast, those earning between $20,000 and $30,000 receive only $599 (see figure 23.4). One reason is that those earning higher incomes are in higher tax brackets. For example, a family in the 40 percent tax bracket gets a subsidy of forty cents for every dollar spent on their health insurance. By contrast, a family in the 15 percent bracket gets a subsidy of only fifteen cents on the dollar.

A uniform subsidy would offer the same tax reduction to everyone who obtains private insurance, and that subsidy should reflect the value our society places on having one more person insured. But what is that value?

Characteristic No. 3: The Revealed Social Value of Insurance Is the Amount We Spend on Free Care for the Uninsured

How do we know how much it is worth collectively for a given individual to insure? An empirically verifiable number is at hand, so long as we're willing to accept the political system as dispositive. It's the amount we expect to spend (from public and private sources) on free care for that person when he or she is uninsured.

To continue with the Texas example, if society is spending $1,000 per year on free care for the uninsured, on the average, we should be willing to offer $1,000 (say, in the form of a tax credit) to everyone who obtains private insurance. Failure to subsidize private insurance as generously as we subsidize free care encourages people to choose the latter.

One reason this principle is not generally understood is that many people think the uninsured are uncared for. In fact, they are not. They are simply participating in a different kind of health care system. As noted earlier, uninsured adults in Dallas County typically seek health care through the emergency room at Parkland Hospital. Uninsured children are typically treated next door, in the emergency room of Children's Medical Center.

Think of the system that provides these services as "safety net insurance," and note that reliance on the safety net is not as valuable to patients as ordinary private insurance, other things being equal. The privately insured patient has more choices of doctors and hospital facilities. Further, safety net care is probably much less efficient (e.g., using emergency rooms to provide care that is more economical in a free-standing clinic). As a result, per dollar spent the privately insured patient probably gets more care and better care.

Characteristic No. 4: The Penalties Paid by the Uninsured Should Be Used to Compensate Those Who Provide Free Care to the Uninsured

What should be done with the penalties collected from people who choose to remain uninsured? They should be used to compensate providers who give free care to the uninsured, no more and no less.[14]

As noted above, under the current system the uninsured pay higher taxes because they do not enjoy the tax relief given to those who have employer-provided insurance. These higher taxes are a "fine" for being uninsured. The problem is the extra taxes paid are simply lumped in with other revenues collected by the U.S. Treasury in Washington, D.C., while the expense of delivering free care falls to local doctors and hospitals.

Under an ideal system, the government would offer every individual a subsidy. If the individual obtained private insurance, the subsidy would be realized in the form of lower taxes (say, in the form of a tax credit). If the individual chose to remain uninsured, the subsidy would be sent to a safety net agency in his or her community (see figure 23.5a). Such an arrangement is a system under which the uninsured as a group pay for their own free care. The very act of turning down a tax credit by choosing not to insure would impose on the uninsured taxes exactly equal to the average cost of free care given annually to the uninsured (see figure 23.5b).[15]

FIGURE 23-5a

The $1,000 Federal Guarantee

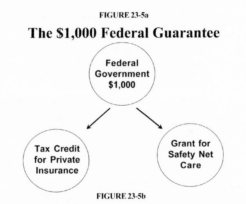

FIGURE 23-5b

The Marginal Effect of Choosing to be Uninsured

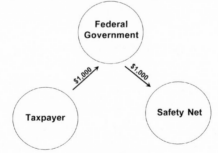

FIGURE 23-5c

The Marginal Effect of Choosing to be Insured

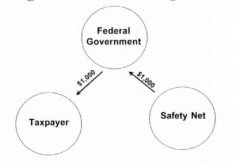

Characteristic No. 5: The Subsidies for the Insured Should, at the Margin, Be Funded by Reducing Spending on Free Care for the Uninsured

How should we fund subsidies for those who choose to move from being uninsured to insured? The answer: at the margin, the subsidy should be funded by the reduction in expected free care that person would have consumed if uninsured, no more and no less.

Suppose everyone in Dallas County chose to obtain private insurance, relying, say, on a refundable $1,000 federal income tax credit to pay the premiums. Dallas County no longer would need to spend $1,000 per person on the uninsured. All of the money that previously funded safety net medical care could be used to fund the private insurance premiums (see figure 23.5c).

How could this scheme be implemented? Since much of the safety net expenditure already consists of federal funds, the federal government could use its share to fund private insurance tax credits instead. For the remainder, the federal government could reduce block grants to Texas for Medicaid and other programs. This arrangement is a system in which people who leave the social safety net and obtain private insurance furnish the funding needed to pay their private insurance premiums, at least at the margin. They do this by allowing public authorities to reduce safety net spending by an amount exactly equal to the private insurance tax subsidy.[16]

Characteristic No. 6: Subsidies for Being Insured Should Be Determined Independently of How the Insurance Is Purchased

The American health care system is largely an employer-based system; more than 90 percent of people with health insurance obtain it from an employer. In recent years many have questioned the wisdom of having employers choose health plans for their employees. Interest in a personal and portable insurance has increased, and many individuals would prefer to take their insurance with them as they change jobs and have employers make defined-contribution premium payments to the plans their employees choose.

These issues should be resolved in the marketplace, rather than by the tax-writing committees of the U.S. Congress.

Figure 23.6 shows that a typical middle-income family with employer provided coverage gets a tax subsidy equal to almost half the cost of insurance. By contrast, families who purchase their own insurance get virtually no relief under the tax law. An ideal system would give the same tax relief, regardless of how the insurance is purchased (see figure 23.7). If the playing field were level under tax law, the employer's role would be determined through competition and choice.

FIGURE 23-6

Federal and State Tax
Subsidies for Private Insurance

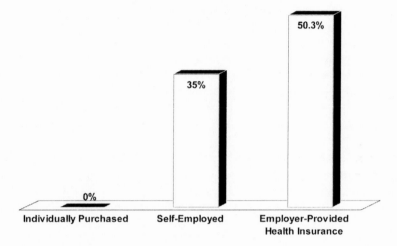

Note: Assumes taxpayer is in the 28 percent federal income tax bracket, faces a 15.3 percent
payroll (FICA) tax and a 7 percent state and local income tax.

FIGURE 23-7

Government Neutrality toward
How Health Insurance Is Purchased

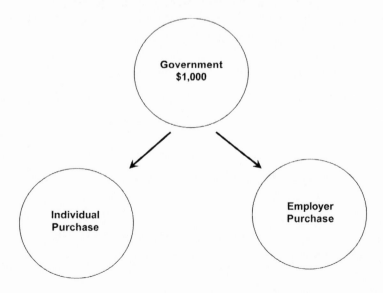

Characteristic No. 7: The Optimal Number of Uninsured Is Not Zero

The goal of health insurance reform is not to get everyone insured. Indeed, everyone is already in a loose sense insured. Instead, the goal is to reach a point at which we are socially indifferent about whether one more person obtains private insurance as an alternative to relying on the social safety net. That is the point at which the marginal cost (in terms of subsidy) to the remaining members of society of the last person we induce to insure is equal to the marginal benefit to the remaining members of society (in terms of the reduction in cost of free care). Once we satisfy this condition, it follows that the number of people who remain uninsured is optimal, and that number is not zero.

This is achieved by taking the average amount spent on free care and making it available for the purchase of private insurance. In our example, the government guarantees that $1,000 is available, depending on the choice of insurance system. From a policy perspective, we are indifferent about the choice people make.

Characteristic No. 8: The Principles of Reform Apply with Equal Force to All Citizens, Regardless of Income

None of the first six points is in any way dependent for its validity on the income of the person who elects to be insured or uninsured. As a practical matter, one could argue that the high-income uninsured are likely to pay more out-of-pocket (get less free care) than the low-income uninsured, and therefore their reward/penalty should be smaller. Against that is the observation that high-income people (because of greater sophistication) are more adept overall at spending other people's money once they enter the health care system.

Waiving these considerations, a $100,000-a-year family can generate hospital bills it cannot pay almost as easily as a $30,000-a-year family. Thus our social interest in whether someone is insured is largely independent of income. For this reason as well as practical considerations, the tax credit should be independent of income.[17]

Characteristic No. 9: Health Insurance Subsidies Need Not Add to Budgetary Outlays

A common misconception is that health insurance reform costs money. For example, if health insurance for forty million people costs $1,000 a person, some conclude that the government would need to spend an additional $40 billion a year to get the job done. But we already spend $40 billion or more on free care for the uninsured, and if all forty million uninsured suddenly became insured they would—in that act—free up the $40 billion from the social safety net.

At $1.5 trillion a year, there is no reason to believe our health care system is spending too little money. To the contrary, attempting to insure the uninsured by spending more money would have the perverse effect of contributing to health care inflation. As Gene Steuerle has shown, we can simply make some portion of people's tax liability contingent on proof of insurance.[18] Getting all the incentives right may involve shifting around a lot of money (i.e., reducing subsidies that are currently too large and increasing subsidies that are too small), but it need not add to budgetary outlays.

For families who already pay substantial federal income taxes, the trick is to make some portion of tax liability contingent on proof of insurance. For example, the child credit (originally $500 per child, scheduled to rise to $1,000) could be tied to proof of insurance. Families that fail to provide proof would lose the credit and pay an additional $1,000 per child in taxes. Similarly, $1,000 of the personal exemption could be tied to proof of insurance.

Families who have children and earn between, say, $10,000 and $30,000 a year generally qualify for the Earned Income Tax Credit (EITC). Even though they owe no income tax, these families can complete a tax return and get a "refund" of as much as $3,000 or $4,000 per year from the Treasury. The payments also could be contingent on proof of insurance, including enrollment in Medicaid, S-CHIP, an employer plan or a privately purchased plan.

Characteristic No. 10: The Federal Government's Role Should Remain Strictly Financial

Currently, the federal government "spends" more than $141 billion a year on tax subsidies for employer-provided insurance. However, the tax code says almost nothing about what features a health insurance plan must have in order to qualify for a tax subsidy.[19] Insurance purchased commercially, around two-thirds of the total, is regulated by the state governments. The federal tax subsidy applies to whatever plans state governments allow.[20]

In this sense, the federal role is strictly financial. The current tax break is based solely on the number of dollars taxpayers spend on health insurance, not on the features of the health plans themselves.

This practice is sensible and should be continued. Aside from an interest in encouraging catastrophic insurance, there is no social reason why government at any level should dictate the content of health insurance plans. To continue our example, the role of the federal government should be to insure that $1,000 is available. It should leave the particulars of the insurance contract to the market and the decisions about safety net health care to local citizens and their elected representatives.

IMPLEMENTING REFORM

Reform of the U.S. health care system is less complicated than it at first might appear. The building blocks of an ideal system are already in place. The federal government already generously subsidizes private health insurance as well as safety net care. The main problem of the current system is its perverse incentives.

One could reasonably argue that government is doing more harm than good, that a laissez faire policy would be better than what we have now. Nonetheless, if government is going to be involved in a major way in our health care system we should act quickly to replace perverse incentives with neutral ones. In particular,

- At a minimum, government policy should be neutral between private insurance and the social safety net—never spending more on free care for the uninsured than it spends to encourage the purchase of private insurance.
- Government policy also should be neutral between individual and employer purchase, allowing the role of the employer to be determined by individual choice and competition in the market place.

If we applied these two principles and no others, we would go a long way toward creating an ideal health care system.

NOTES

1. Robert J. Mills and Shailesh Bhandari, "Health Insurance Coverage in the United States: 2002," Current Population Reports P60-223, U.S. Census Bureau, U.S. Department of Commerce, September 2003; Bureau of the Census, "Health Insurance Coverage—1993," Statistical Brief, SB/94-28, U.S. Census Bureau, U.S. Department of Commerce, October 1994.

2. John C. Goodman, "Characteristics of an Ideal Health Care System," National Center for Policy Analysis, Policy Report No. 242, April 2001.

3. Jill M. Yegian et al., "The Nonpoor Uninsured in California, 1998," *Health Affairs* 19, no. 4 (July/August 2000) 171–77.

4. Melinda L. Schriver and Grace-Marie Arnett, "What States Can Teach Congress about Health Care Regulation," Heritage Foundation, Backgrounder No. 2107, July 23, 1998.

5. John C. Goodman and Gerald L. Musgrave, "Freedom of Choice in Health Insurance," National Center for Policy Analysis, Policy Report No. 134, November 1988.

6. Frank A. Sloan and Christopher J. Conover, "Effects of State Reforms on Health Insurance Coverage of Adults," *Inquiry* 3 (1998): 280–93.

7. Gail A. Jensen and Michael A. Morrisey, "Mandated Benefit Laws and Employer-Sponsored Health Insurance," *Health Insurance Association of America,* January 1999.

8. A group health plan can exclude preexisting medical conditions from coverage for no more than twelve months except when individuals enroll after the open enrollment period. Exclusions on the latter can apply for eighteen months.

9. Jack Hadley and John Holahan, "How Much Medical Care Do The Uninsured Use, And Who Pays For It?" *Health Affairs* (February 12, 2003) (Web Exclusive W3-66).

10. "Hospitals Uncompensated Have Expenses Not Keeping Pace with Per Capita Spending, "Health Care Financing and Organization: News and Progress (March 2000), 5–6.

11. "Indigent Care: Insurers Are 'Overburdened and Threadbare,'" *American Health Line* (March 31, 2000) reporting the conclusions of *American Health Safety Net: Intact but Endangered*, Marion Ein Lewin and Stuart Altman, eds. (Washington, D.C.: National Academy Press, 2000).

12. Lewin Group estimates using the Health Benefits Simulation Model.

13. An ideal subsidy would not distort decisions at the margin. People would be able to choose on a level playing field between health care and nonhealth care and between health care today and health care tomorrow. See Mark V. Pauly and John C. Goodman, "Tax Credits for Health Insurance and Medical Savings Accounts," *Health Affairs* 14, no. 1 (Spring 1995): 126–39.

14. Low-income families who do not otherwise owe any federal income tax will not literally be paying their own way. But in forgoing, say, a $1,000 refundable tax credit they will be making a decision that allows the $1,000 to be deposited in a local safety net.

15. To our knowledge, this idea was first proposed in John C. Goodman and Gerald L. Musgrave, *Patient Power: Solving America's Health Care Crisis* (Washington, D.C.: Cato Institute, 1992). Also, see Lynn Etheredge, "A Flexible Benefits Tax Credit for Health Insurance and More," *Health Affairs,* special Internet-only publication, available at www.healthaffairs.org/2003Etheredge.pdf.

16. Some patients may be high cost. In a private insurance market, insurers will not agree to insure someone for $1,000 if his or her expected cost of care is, say, $5,000. But if the safety net agency expects a $5,000 savings as a result of the loss of a patient to a private insurer, the agency should be willing to pay up to $5,000 to subsidize the private insurance premium.

17. Society has no reason to care whether Bill Gates is insured. So there could be an income or wealth threshold beyond which the subsidy/penalty system does not apply. However, as a practical matter so few individuals would qualify for an exemption that uniform treatment is administratively attractive.

18. C. Eugene Steuerle, "Child Credits: Opportunity at the Door," Urban Institute, 1997. Although Steuerle does not say so, one way to insure is to self-insure. So proof of insurance could include evidence of a self-funded Health Savings Account.

19. The exceptions are mandated maternity coverage, federal mandates requiring a forty-eight-hour hospital stay after a well-baby delivery if requested by patient and physician, and mandated mental health parity.

20. M. Susan Marquis and Stephen H. Long, "Recent Trends in Self-Insured Employer Health Plans," *Health Affairs* 18, no. 3 (May/June 1999): 161–66.

Chapter Twenty-four

Designing Ideal Health Insurance

The modern era has inherited two models of health insurance: the fee-for-service model and the HMO model. Neither is appropriate to the Information Age.

Both models assume that (1) the amount of sickness is limited and largely outside the control of the insureds, (2) methods of treating illness are limited and well defined, and (3) because of patient ignorance and asymmetry of information, treatment decisions will always be filtered by physicians, based on their own knowledge and experience or clinical practice guidelines.

However, an explosion of technological innovation and the rapid diffusion of knowledge about the potential of medical science to diagnose and treat disease have rendered these assumptions obsolete. In this chapter, we briefly outline the type of insurance we believe would emerge if we rely on markets, rather than regulators, to solve our problems.

WHY TECHNOLOGICAL CHANGE AND THE DIFFUSION OF KNOWLEDGE HAVE MADE TRADITIONAL HEALTH INSURANCE MODELS OBSOLETE

Although the HMO model is often viewed as the more contemporary, it is actually the less compatible with the changes the medical marketplace is undergoing. The traditional HMO model is fundamentally based on patient ignorance. The basic idea is a simple one: make health care free at the point of consumption and control costs by having physicians ration care, eliminating options that are judged "unnecessary" or at least not "cost-effective."

But this model works only as long as patients are willing to accept their doctor's opinion. And that only works as long as patients are unaware of other (possibly more expensive) options.

As we argued in the Introduction, we could spend our entire gross domestic product on health care in useful ways. In fact, we could probably spend the entire GDP on diagnostic tests alone—without ever treating a real disease. The information reality is that patients are becoming as informed as their doctors—not about how to practice medicine, but about how the practice of medicine can benefit them. Combine the potential of modern medicine to benefit patients with a general awareness of these benefits and zero out-of-pocket payments, and the HMO model is simply courting disaster. The fee-for-service model is only a slight improvement. It tries to control demand by introducing deductibles and copays. But even it offers strong incentives for patients to overconsume health care.

Some believe that managed care can solve these problems. They are wrong. Imagine grocery insurance that allows you to buy all the groceries you need; but as you stroll down the supermarket aisle, you are confronted with a team of bureaucrats, prepared to argue over your every purchase. Would anyone want to buy such a policy? Traditional health insurance isn't designed to work much better.

Accordingly, we propose a new approach. It combines an old concept, casualty insurance, with two relatively new concepts: universal HSAs (to control demand) and a proliferation of focused factories (to control supply).

DESIGNING AN IDEAL HEALTH INSURANCE PLAN

Let's begin by wiping the slate clean. Imagine you could get together with 999 other people and create an insurance plan just for 1,000 people. The 1,000 people are not alike. Some are old; some are young. Some are male; some are female. Some are in good health; some are not. Given these and other differences, how can you design a plan that all would want to join?

In answering this question, forget the normal insurance industry bureaucracy. Forget state and federal regulations. Forget federal tax law. Forget everything else that would pose an artificial impediment to achieving the ideal. You're on your own. You must design a plan that will come closest to meeting your needs and those of your colleagues. What follows is a discussion of some inevitable problems and some proposed solutions. We hope this thought experiment will point to how insurance markets would evolve if left free to do so.[1]

Terms of Entry

One of the first decisions you must make is: what premiums should be charged to people when they join the insurance pool? No matter what benefits you decide to include in the plan, you have to collect enough premiums to cover all the costs. So how much should each person pay? We have a suggestion that not only will solve this problem, but also will avoid many others. In fact, failure to follow our suggestion on this issue will virtually guarantee that your group will not agree on anything else. Our suggestion is this: each person should pay a premium equal to the expected health care costs he or she adds to the 1,000-person pool. If individual A will add $1,000, the right premium for A is $1,000. If B's expected costs are $5,000, B should pay $5,000. If C's expected costs are $10,000, C should pay $10,000.

What if the premium is so high for some people that they cannot afford to pay it? Then either they will be left out of the pool or others must make a charitable contribution on their behalf. Since all agreements are voluntary in this imagined scenario, coercion is not an option. Politicians usually try to "solve" the problem by keeping the premium artificially low for people with high health care costs. But if some people are undercharged, others must be overcharged.

People who are overcharged will want less coverage than they otherwise would, and those who are undercharged will want more. If we want people to make economically rational decisions, they must be charged a premium that makes the expected benefit of their additional coverage equal to its expected cost.

Terms of Renewal

At the end of an insurance period of, say, one year, on what terms should people be allowed to renew? Should those whose health has deteriorated be charged more? Should people whose health has improved be charged less?

Insurance can be compared to gambling. Our decision to charge each entrant in the pool a premium equal to his or her expected costs makes the gamble a "fair" bet for all. But changing premiums based on changes in health status would be like changing the rules after throwing the dice. It would defeat the purpose of insurance, which is to transfer risk to others. Therefore, a reasonable rule is to raise or lower everyone's premium at renewal time, based on whether the whole group's costs have been more or less than expected. Those who got sick and generated high medical costs after joining the pool would not be penalized and would get the full value of the insurance.

Such a rule is broadly characteristic of the market for individual insurance. At the time of initial enrollment, people may be charged different premiums, based on age, sex and perhaps health status. But once in a plan, no one can be expelled from it or charged an extra premium because his or her health deteriorates. Renewal is guaranteed, and if premiums are increased, they must be increased proportionately for everyone.

The small group market now operates quite differently in most states. A firm's premiums are readjusted annually, based not on the experience of the larger group with which the firm's employees have been pooled, but on the firm's employees' own experience over the previous year. In effect, it's as though every firm's employees were kicked out of the pool at the end of the year and allowed to reenter only if they pay new premiums based on the changes in their expected health costs. Subject to regulatory constraints, in the small group market people can buy insurance only one year at a time. If this practice applied to life insurance, everyone's premium would be reassessed annually, and rates for those diagnosed with cancer or AIDS during the previous year would be astronomical. Such a practice would virtually destroy the market for life insurance.[2] Small wonder that small group health insurance markets are in perpetual crisis.

The features of the individual market described above come closest to emulating what most economists would consider a free market for health insurance, although the market is far from perfect. By contrast, the features of the small group market are almost totally the product of unwise public policies—federal tax law, federal regulations and state regulations. Not surprisingly, this market has generated the most frequent complaints, particularly from small business owners. Unfortunately most states try to deal with the problem by piling on more regulations rather than by confronting its cause.

Third-Party Insurance versus Self-Insurance

The decision about what services to cover is closely related to the decision about how to allocate financial responsibility. For reasons that will become clear, the latter question needs to be addressed first. As noted above, recent changes in federal law allow deposits to HSAs to receive the same tax advantage as employer-paid premiums. Prior to that change, federal tax law encouraged people to give all their health dollars to third-party payers. But under neutral federal tax law, which services would we choose to pay directly and which would we insure for? That is, what medical costs would we want the pool to pay for, and which ones would we want to pay from our own resources?

Any time people transfer their resources to an insurance pool, there are two negative consequences (increased cost, at least for the group as a whole, and decreased autonomy) and one positive (reduced risk). The problem is to assure that the reduction in risk is worth the extra premium we must pay to obtain it. Our imaginary insurance pool faces the same problems as every other insurance scheme. Any time insurance pays a medical bill, the incentives of the patient are distorted. All of us tend to overconsume when someone else is paying the bill, and this tendency, which economists call the problem of "moral hazard," raises costs. To counteract the tendency, we will want to consider some of the techniques of managed care. But these techniques will restrict our choices, reduce our autonomy and perhaps reduce the quality of the care we get. Even if the quality is not diminished, administering the techniques will be costly.

Thus, no matter how well the plan is designed, for the group as a whole the cost of medical care will be higher than it would be if individuals simply purchased the same care on their own. Presumably, the higher costs are worthwhile if we enjoy enough reduction in risk. But at what point does the price we're paying for risk reduction become too high? Specifically, when is it worthwhile to transfer risk to a pool and when does it make better sense to self-insure by putting funds into an account we own and control? Three general questions can help us arrive at an answer:

1. Is the medical service to be purchased prompted by a risky event or by an individual preference?
2. Is the price of transferring risk to a third party high or low?
3. Does the failure to obtain a service or the purchase of an inappropriate service potentially create costs for others in the pool?

The first question relates to the terms under which people obtain health care services. People differ in their attitudes toward medical care. They also differ in their levels of aversion to risk. Take diagnostic tests for the detection of cancer. As noted above, the more frequent the tests, the higher the cost. But medical science cannot tell us how frequent such exams should be.[3] That is largely a value judgment, and people's values differ. In general, such exams are not prompted by a risky event; they are influenced by individual preferences.

As a general rule, the more expenditures depend on personal choices rather than external events, the greater will be the problem of moral hazard. This consideration suggests we should encourage individuals to purchase directly most diagnostic tests and most forms of preventive medicine.

The second question reinforces this conclusion. Transferring the risk of cancer treatment to an insurance pool is relatively low-cost. For each dollar of exposure transferred, the extra premium is only a few pennies. On the other hand, transferring diagnostic testing to an insurance pool is relatively high-cost. For each dollar of exposure transferred, the extra premium is a large part of that dollar. So the payoff for using insurance to cover cancer treatment is high, while the payoff for covering cancer detection is low.

The third question is whether the medical consequences of one's decision will generate costs for other members of the pool. Take immunization for childhood diseases for example. Studies show that these procedures pay for themselves by avoiding future health care costs that are greater than the costs of the vaccinations.[4] This implies that members of an insurance pool have an economic self-interest in seeing that all children covered by the pool are vaccinated. It may make economic sense for the pool to pay for vaccinations, thereby incurring more cost than self-pay would generate, or to require that members obtain them, thereby reducing autonomy.

Closely related to the problem created by the failure to obtain a desirable service is the problem created by the purchase of the wrong service. Suppose our plan has a $3,000 deductible and a member is diagnosed with cancer. Under this arrangement, the patient would pay the first $3,000 of treatment costs and presumably would make his or her own decisions about how to spend the $3,000. But that $3,000 of decision making could have a large impact on later treatment costs, and bad decisions early on could generate larger subsequent costs for the group. Such considerations may create a presumption in favor of paying for all treatment costs from the pool in cases where the entire treatment regime promises to be expensive.[5]

Table 24.1 summarizes the case for a division between individual payment for medical services and third-party payment. Third-party payment for every medical service is potentially very wasteful. Such waste can be controlled only by invasive, expensive third-party oversight of individual medical care consumption. Such control necessarily interferes in the doctor-patient relationship. Some people may prefer this sacrifice of autonomy, and that may explain why there has always been a market for the traditional HMO. But many people will prefer self-pay and self-control, especially where no real reduction in financial risk is achieved by transferring control to a third-party payer.

Figure 24.1 shows that even after taking into account each of the general rules in table 24.1, some health services may not neatly fit into unambiguous "self-pay" or "third-party pay" categories. Ideal health plans might have considerable discretion, therefore, and how they exercise it would depend on their members' preferences. What is important is to recognize that in the ideal insurance arrangement, some decisions will be individual while others will be collective.

TABLE 24-1

General Rules

Individual Choice	*Collective Choice*
1. No risky medical event.	1. Risky medical event.
2. Price of third-party insurance is high.	2. Price of third-party insurance is low.
3. Exercise of choice creates no externalities.	3. Exercise of choice creates risks for others.

Financing Mechanism for Self-Insurance: HSAs

A common objection to individual control is that people will not always make wise decisions. But in our imaginary pool, everyone must voluntarily agree to the design of the plan, so we cannot entirely escape individual choice and preference. In addition, even with the most comprehensive coverage, indi-

FIGURE 24-1

Appropriate Division of
Financial Responsibility

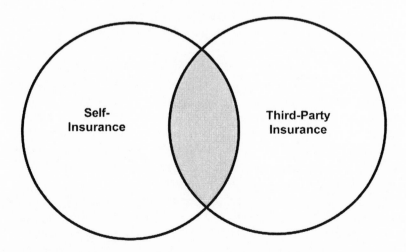

Self-
Insurance

Third-Party
Insurance

viduals must make decisions about when to see a doctor and whether to purchase nonprescription drugs. So even if a patient wanted to turn all decisions
over to someone else, that would be impossible. A more sophisticated objection is that most medical expenditures tend to be irregular, and are hard for
people living from paycheck-to-paycheck to incorporate into a budget.

One answer to this objection is the HSA. As described above, many employers make monthly deposits to accounts from which their employees can
pay expenses not covered by the employer's health plan.[6] Money not spent
for medical care must remain in the account until the end of the insurance
period, usually one year, after which the employee can withdraw it and use
it for other purposes.[7] HSAs make individual self-insurance workable for
families who otherwise might find direct payment too burdensome. But how
should such accounts be designed in conjunction with third-party insurance
coverage?

Implications for HSA Design

The left side of figure 24.2 illustrates the most common design of HSAs in
employer plans. The plan pays all costs above a deductible of, say, $3,000.
The HSA deposit in this example is $2,000. Thus, the employee pays the
first $2,000 of medical expenses from the HSA and the next $1,000 is paid
out of pocket. Any remaining costs are paid by the plan.[8] Note that with
freedom comes added responsibility. In current employer plans, individuals
are usually free to use their HSA funds to purchase noncovered services. So,
an employee might spend all of his or her HSA account on chiropractor
services—even if these services are not covered by the plan and the payments do not count toward the deductible. An employee could exhaust the
HSA funds on noncovered services and risk having to pay the entire deductible out of pocket.

However, HSAs designed in this way are not necessarily ideal. The above
considerations imply that the design pictured on the right side of figure 24.2
is preferable. Under this design, the plan pays the first dollar for some treatments, while leaving the insured free to pay even higher amounts for some
services than in the illustration on the left. Indeed, one way to think about the
diagram at left is to see it as a special case of the diagram at right—one which
would be voluntarily chosen only if all the considerations in table 24.1 were
appropriately resolved by an across-the-board deductible.

The diagram on the right has a further advantage: it can fit into existing
managed care plans. One problem these plans have in maintaining member
satisfaction was summarized by Alain Enthoven in a well-publicized letter to
then governor Pete Wilson of California.[9] Enthoven described a woman who

FIGURE 24-2

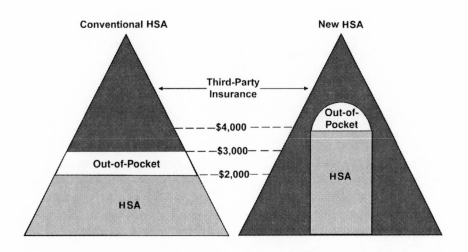

was angry at her HMO doctor because he refused her a "medically unneces-sary" sonogram. Enthoven surmised that if she'd had to pay fifty dollars out of her own pocket for the service, she would have thanked her doctor for sav-ing her the expense. This and other incidents have convinced Enthoven, who has been wedded for years to the concept of the first-dollar coverage, that pa-tient out-of-pocket pay is essential to make managed care work.

Interestingly, there is one place in the world where the diagram on the right has become a reality—South Africa. Since 1993 virtually all major forms of insurance have been competing on a level playing field (HMOs, PPOs and MSAs) partly due to liberal insurance regulations and partly due to a favor-able ruling from the South African equivalent of the IRS. Anyone with an idea on how to design a better health insurance plan has been free to try. And dur-ing the decade of the 1990s MSA plans have captured more than half of the market for private health insurance. Under federal law, a tax-free HSA for Americans must have at least a $1,000 deductible for individuals and $2,000 for families and applies to all services—drugs, physician care, hospital care, and so forth. South African HSAs are more flexible. The typical plan has the first-dollar insurance coverage for most hospital procedures—on the theory that within hospitals patients have little opportunity to exercise choices. On the other hand, a high deductible (about $1,200) applies to "discretionary ex-penses," including most services delivered in doctors' offices.[10]

South Africa's more flexible approach also allows more sensible drug cov-erage. While the high deductible applies to most drugs for ordinary patients, a typical plan pays from the first dollar for drugs for diabetes, asthma and other chronic conditions. The theory: it's not smart to encourage patients to skimp on drugs that prevent more-expensive-to-treat conditions from developing.

The Design of Third-Party Payment

One of the fastest-growing health insurance products toward the close of the last decade was the point-of-service (POS) option. This option has been popular because employees complained about the restrictiveness of closed networks. Yet, analysts say that POS options can raise the cost of health insurance by 11 percent or more.[11] It's as though people flock to managed care plans to take advantage of their low premiums, then demand options that undermine the ability of the plans to keep costs down.

The approach summarized in table 24.1 points to a partial solution. The reason out-of-network doctors cost more, even when paid the same fees as in-network physicians, is that they are likely to order more tests and generate the use of more ancillary services. But this would be of much less concern if third-party payment were restricted largely to curative services and patients paid with their HSA funds for diagnostic services.

The problem of how to control curative costs without unduly restricting patient choice or endangering quality remains. A possible solution is a variant on an old idea: a fee schedule. From time to time, the insurance industry has flirted with plans that pay doctors a set fee for various services. If patients selected doctors who charge more, they paid the difference out of pocket. In modern medicine, we know that the doctor's fee is only one part of a complex array of costs a doctor can generate. So controlling the physician's fee isn't enough. But why not fix the plan's cost for an entire treatment regime? Suppose a patient is diagnosed with cancer, and the health plan normally would contract to pay a fixed fee to a medical facility to cover all costs.[12] If the plan could be assured that this fixed fee were its maximum exposure, the plan would have no economic interest in restricting the patient's choices. It could, for example, allow the patient to go to an alternative provider and pay more, if needed, out of pocket or from an HSA. In this way, the plan controls its costs and patients still exercise choice; the exercise of choice puts pressure on the plan to maintain quality in its own preferred medical facility.

The decision to take the plan's money and seek treatment elsewhere need not be made once and for all. For chronic conditions, it could be reaffirmed annually. Take diabetes. Because traditional care for diabetes has been less than optimal,[13] many patients and doctors have long maintained that patients (with the help of a physician) can manage diabetes more efficiently than managed care can.[14] Why not let them try? The health plan might make an annual deposit to the patient's HSA and shift the entire year's financial responsibility to the patient. If there were concern that the funds might be wasted, the health plan could hold the account and monitor it. An example of the range of possibilities is again provided by South Africa. Discovery Health (one of the largest sellers of MSA plans there) allows its diabetic patients the opportunity to enroll in a special diabetes management program. Under the arrangement, Discovery pays the program about seventy-five dollars per month, while patients pay another twenty-five dollars from their MSA accounts. Discovery is considering handling many other chronic diseases in the same way.

The Casualty Insurance Model

To appreciate where this line of thinking might lead, compare casualty insurance with traditional health insurance. After an automobile accident, a claims adjuster inspects the damage, agrees on a price and writes the car owner a check. Hail damage to a home's roof is handled in the same way under a homeowner's policy. In both cases, the insured is free to make his or her own decisions about paying for damage repair. In contrast, traditional health insurance is based on the idea that insurers should pay not for conditions, but for medical care. That health insurers rejected the casualty model is not surprising. After all, Blue Cross was started by hospitals for the purpose of insuring that hospital bills would be paid. Blue Shield was started by doctors to ensure that doctor fees would be paid.[15] Had auto insurance been developed by auto repair shops, they also would have rejected the casualty model.

We are not suggesting that we give the insured complete freedom of choice. Paying people for a condition and allowing them to forego health care and spend the money on pleasure may not be in the self-interest of a health insurance pool, because an untreated condition today could develop into a new and more expensive-to-treat condition later on.[16] We are suggesting that if people were largely free to make their own treatment choices and the market were free to meet their needs, health insurance would take a major step in the direction of the casualty model.

Covered Services

One of the most contentious issues in health politics today concerns the services health insurers must cover. Special interests have persuaded state legislatures to require insurers to cover a vast array of costly services, whether or not those buying the insurance want to pay for coverage for those services.[17] In our hypothetical plan, however, these special interests get no voice. Only the 1,000 enrollees count. That said, traditional insurance has made a lot of arbitrary distinctions that an ideal plan need not make. For example, traditional insurance paid for treatment of back problems by an M. D., but not a chiropractor. It paid for mental health services provided by a psychiatrist, but not a psychologist. The rationale was partly a misplaced attempt to save money, but it also reflected the physicians' interest in promoting insurance that pays for the services of medical doctors rather than the individuals' interest in protection against catastrophic costs.

The casualty model of insurance helps solve this problem. Health plans could control costs and give patients greater freedom to choose among competing providers at the same time. Coupled with the idea that people should pay their full cost when entering a health plan and that medical consumption decisions not arising from a risky event should be paid by the individual from an MSA, our ideal health plan should make coverage decisions a lot easier.

Terms of Exit

Recall that insurance contracts in the individual market are almost always guaranteed renewable. Once in an insurance pool, people are entitled to remain there indefinitely and pay the same premiums others pay, regardless of changes in their health status. That commitment is completely one-sided, however. The insurer makes an indefinite commitment to the members, but the members are free to leave the pool at any time.

This one-way commitment creates the following problem. New insurance pools attract mainly healthy people because insurers tend to deny coverage, or attach exclusions and riders limiting the coverage of persons who are already sick (a process known as "medical underwriting"). As time passes, some enrollees get sick and the premium paid by all must be increased to cover the cost of their care. Thus, mature insurance pools will almost always charge higher premiums than young pools. This gives healthy people an incentive to leave the mature pool. By switching to a young pool, healthy people can escape high premiums. But this option is not open to the sick members of the mature pool. If they try to switch, the new pool will either deny them coverage or charge them a higher premium because of their medical condition. As a result, it is not unusual in the individual market to find an insurer providing the same coverage, but charging vastly different premiums, depending on the age of the pool. Members of a mature pool, for example, might pay $1,000 a month or more for their coverage, while entrants into a young pool might pay only a few hundred dollars. Clearly, these are not the features of an ideal insurance system.

A possible solution is to make the long-term commitment apply both ways. In return for an indefinite commitment on the part of the insurer, members would commit to the pool for a period of, say, three, four or five years. This does not mean that people would remain stuck in a plan they wished to leave. It does mean that leaving the pool would require the consent of the pool. For example, if a healthy member left high-cost plan A to join low-cost plan B, B would compensate A for its loss. Conversely, if a sick member left A to join B, A would compensate B to take the member and pay for the higher expected cost of care.[18] In this model, recontracting is always possible, but only the type of recontracting that leaves everybody better off.[19]

Moreover, in the ideal system described here, people would have far less reason to switch insurers because their pool would be providing mainly financial (insurance) services rather than health care. A member would not need to switch from plan A to plan B to see a particular doctor or gain a higher quality of care.

Can Markets Develop Ideal Health Insurance Plans?

The ideas outlined here are merely suggestive. We do not expect individuals to develop their own health plans. That's what competition and markets are supposed to do. Entrepreneurs are supposed to innovate and experiment to find the products people want to buy. But intrusive regulations aside, can we rely on the market to achieve the best result?

Patients as Buyers of Health Care

As we saw in chapter 13, one objection to individuals paying directly for most diagnostic and preventive services is that they would not get the lowest price or find the highest quality. But anecdotal evidence suggests that uninsured individuals, spending their own money, get as good a discount as do large buyers.[20] Even if this were not true, there's no reason why the health plan itself cannot negotiate discounts for its members, even if the members spend their own money when they receive the services.

The issue of quality is a bit more difficult. But the solution is not the first-dollar managed care for every service. Suppose that as part of its HMO network, Blue Cross set up primary care clinics for its members. Blue Cross asserts that these clinics deliver high-quality, cost-effective care. If the assertion is true, why limit the care to the HMO members? Why not allow anyone to enter the clinic and pay out of pocket for the same services? This has already happened in cities across the country—proving that fee-for-service payment and cost-effective care are not inconsistent, provided incentives are not distorted in other ways. There's no reason why a health plan should object to patients directly contracting for their health care as long as the plan's own costs do not go up. Indeed, the plan itself could provide consulting and other buying services to help patients make wise choices.

Centers of Excellence and Focused Factories

Can there be a workable market for expensive, curative services—with patients paying the bill? In some places there already is. Managed care advocates often point to the Mayo clinic as an example of cost-effective medicine. They ignore the fact that most of Mayo's customers are fee-for-service patients. What Harvard University professor Regina Herzlinger calls "focused factories," providing highly efficient, specialized care, are becoming a reality.[21] These health care businesses deliver lower prices, lower mortality rates, shorter stays and higher patient satisfaction.

For example, the Johns Hopkins Breast Center is a focused factory for mastectomies. The Dartmouth-Hitchcock Medical Center in Lebanon, New Hampshire, is a focused factory for heart surgery. The Pediatrix Medical Group, which manages neonatal units and provides pediatric services in twenty-one states, is another example.[22] Focused factories also are cropping up around the country to provide cancer, gynecological and orthopedic services. One spectacular success story is Dr. Bernard Salick, a kidney specialist who has become a millionaire by pioneering a national chain of round-the-clock cancer clinics.

Patients on their own can already take advantage of these emerging markets. Indeed, some focused factories are advertising directly to patients. In a *New York Times Magazine* advertisement, Memorial Sloan-Kettering Cancer Center boasted "the best cancer care anywhere" and described how its specialists saved a life after doctors at other hospitals had given up hope.[23]

The Role of Employers

In the absence of federal tax law, why would employers become involved in their employees' health insurance. There are two reasons why employers might become involved, even with neutral government policies. One is the economies of group buying. Signing one contract for all employees involves less overhead than having agents sell individual insurance household by household. There may be some merit to this argument, but it is a rationale exaggerated by people who focus only on the first-year cost. Under current practice, employer group plans are renegotiated every year, whereas individuals usually stay in their plans for several years. Taking into account all costs over several years, the difference in cost is much less. This, presumably, is why employers rarely get involved in their employees' purchase of automobile or homeowners insurance and play only a minor role in the purchase of life insurance.

A second reason for employers' involvement relates to the adverse selection problem. Medical underwriting—attempting to determine everyone's health status at the point of entry into a plan—is costly. Employer-sponsored group insurance avoids this cost by enrolling everyone—the sick as well as the healthy—at once. Further, group contracts are written in ways that discourage individuals from "gaming" the system by remaining out of the pool while they are healthy and then joining the pool once they get sick. Since in the typical arrangement the employer pays a large share of the premium, employees don't save much by remaining uninsured. In addition, new employees have to make the decision to join the pool on a specified date. Thus, the timing of the decision to insure does not coincide with the timing of illness.

Having acknowledged that there may be good reasons for employers to play a role independent of government policies designed to encourage them to do so, let us also acknowledge that the appropriate role of the employer does not have to be settled by armchair theorists. We can let the market decide. Increasingly, employers are moving away from a defined benefit approach and toward a defined contribution approach. This means that employers make a commitment of x dollars to each employee and their employees make their own insurance choices. Remember, this is the approach taken by the federal government for its employees, by most state and local governments for their employees and by some large private employers, although note the problems with these systems discussed in chapter 22. There is no reason in principle why employers cannot help employees reap the economies of group purchase and avoid the costs of medical underwriting, while at the same time acquiring personal and portable individual coverage.[24]

THE BENEFITS OF IDEAL HEALTH INSURANCE

Three features of ideal health insurance would make it especially superior to the health insurance arrangements that prevail today.

Ideal Health Insurance Is Patient Centered

A large portion of our health care dollars would be placed in accounts that we individually own and control. Patients would pay for the vast majority of medical services from these accounts, and doctors would be free to act as agents for their patients rather than for third-party payers. But because patients would be spending their own money in the medical marketplace, physicians would be encouraged to become financial advisers as well as health advisers. Doctors would compete not just on the basis of quality, but on the basis of value for money.

Ideal health insurance in the treatment of expensive conditions would be patient centered. Rather than have a third party pay every medical bill, insurers would make regular deposits to the HSAs of patients with chronic conditions, leaving them free to choose among competing focused factories for ongoing treatment. Rather than have a third party dictate terms and conditions for the delivery of expensive acute care, patients would be able to draw on a fixed sum of money and get their health needs met at a center of excellence or a focused factory of their own choosing.

Ideal Health Insurance Allows Insurers to Specialize in the Business of Insurance

One of the consequences of the managed care revolution is that insurers have been turned into providers of care. That is, the entity that pays our medical bills is the same entity that delivers our medical care. This development has had three negative consequences.

First, when the businesses of insurance and health care merge, health plans have perverse incentives to deny care. The rash of news stories reporting on the tragic consequences of underprovision of care are testimony to what can go wrong.

Second, when the choice of insurer is also effectively a choice of provider networks, consumers must make decisions that are humanly impossible. Ideally, one should not have to choose a cardiologist until one has a heart problem. One should not have to choose an oncologist until one gets cancer. But in today's market, when you choose your insurer you are at the same time choosing your heart specialist and your cancer specialist, whether you are aware of it or not.

Third, the managed care revolution has delegated to those on the buyers' side of the market (insurers) the responsibility of forcing those on the sellers' side of the market (doctors, hospital administrators, etc.) to deliver care efficiently. In no other market do we depend upon buyers to tell sellers how to produce their product. Undoubtedly, there are good reasons why other markets are not organized this way.

Ideal health insurance, by contrast, allows insurers to specialize in what they do best: manage risk. The supply side of the market would be encouraged to organize into focused factories and adopt other efficient techniques in order to produce high quality for low cost. The market would still be free to combine insurance and health care delivery where the combination makes sense. It may turn out that for such specialized services as cancer care, efficiency warrants specialized insurance products. Ideal health insurance would allow those market developments by providing a mechanism for people to leave one insurance pool and join another (without extra cost) when their health condition changes.

Ideal Health Insurance Is Improved by the Free Flow of Information

Under the current system, consumer information is a threat to the stability and peace of mind of typical HMO personnel. The more patients learn, the more they are likely to demand. Under ideal health insurance, by contrast, accurate consumer information is a positive. The reason is that the insurer and the insured are on the same team, with a similar interest and objective: acquiring good value in a competitive market.

Needless to say, the changes outlined here will require appropriate changes in public policy. Of these, three are particularly important.[25]

First, federal tax law must create a level playing field between third-party insurance and individual self-insurance through HSAs. As noted, the United States has already made a major step in that direction. Individual preference and market competition, not the peculiarities of the tax law, should determine the appropriate division.

Second, federal tax law must create a level playing field between employer purchase and individual purchase of health insurance. Although employers can purchase employee health insurance with before-tax dollars, people who purchase their own insurance get virtually no tax relief and must pay with after-tax dollars. (An exception to this generalization is the self-employed, who get partial tax relief.) Employers may have an important role to play in helping people obtain health insurance, but this role should be determined by the marketplace, not by tax law.

A third important change needs to be implemented at the state level. Many employers would like to move to a defined-contribution approach to employee health insurance. As a result, employees could enter a health insurance pool and stay there—taking their insurance coverage with them as they travel from job to job. Personal and portable health insurance is an idea whose time has come. Yet, virtually every state has made this approach (technically known as "list billing") either illegal or prohibitively impractical.

These changes will not solve our most important health insurance problems. They will create a legal environment in which individuals, their employers and their insurers—pursuing their own interests—are likely to create the institutions they need.

NOTES

1. Although we confine our analysis to health insurance, people in an ideal world would probably be inclined to combine health insurance with other forms of insurance. That is, in an ideal insurance world, coverage probably would include health insurance, disability insurance, long-term care and life insurance.

2. The market would collapse to a market for one-year term insurance; and people with terminal illnesses would essentially become uninsurable.

3. Tammy O. Tengs et al., "Five Hundred Lifesaving Interventions and Their Cost-Effectiveness," *Risk Analysis* 15, no. 3 (June 1995), 369; David M. Eddy, ed., *Common Screening Tests* (Philadelphia: American College of Physicians, 1991).

4. Tengs, "Five-Hundred Lifesaving Interventions," 379.

5. Of course, the plan could then require a second opinion, retesting, and so forth.

6. John C. Goodman, "Medical Savings Accounts: The Private Sector Already Has Them," National Center for Policy Analysis, Brief Analysis No. 105, April 20, 1994.

7. Prior to 2004, such deposits were subject to payroll taxes and income taxes. The exceptions were tax-free MSAs allowed under a federal pilot program for the self-employed and employees of small businesses. However, under the pilot program, year-end withdrawals used for nonmedical purposes faced regular income taxes and a 15 percent penalty. As of 2004, HSAs in principle became available to all nonelderly Americans and withdrawals for nonmedical purposes prior to age sixty-five face income taxes plus a 10 percent penalty. Withdrawals after age sixty-five face no penalty.

8. This structure was actually required by law under the federal pilot program that made MSA deposits tax free for the self-employed and employees of small businesses. See Merrill Matthews, "Medical Savings Account Legislation: The Good, the Bad and the Ugly," National Center for Policy Analysis, Brief Analysis No. 211, August 19, 1996.

9. Letter from Alain Enthoven to Gov. Pete Wilson et al., January 6, 1998.

10. Of course, without some oversight, this reimbursement formula encourages discretionary procedures to relocate to a hospital setting.

11. A mandatory point of service option when combined with a requirement to reimburse at the same rates in and out of the network can raise the cost of health insurance by as much as 11.3 percent. Estimates of M&R for the National Center for Policy Analysis. Cited in Merrill Matthews, "Can We Afford Consumer Protection? An Analysis of the PARCA Bill," National Center for Policy Analysis, NCPA Brief Analysis No. 249, November 24, 1997.

12. Some insurers currently pay providers based on the patient's diagnostic related group (DRG). Medicare pays the same way.

13. Regina E. Herzlinger, *Market Driven Health Care: Who Wins, Who Loses in the Transformation of America's Largest Service Industry* (Reading, Mass.: Addison-Wesley, 1997), 173.

14. For a survey of the efficacy of self-monitoring, see A. Faas, F. G. Schellevis and J. T. Van Eijk, "The Efficacy of Self-Monitoring of Blood Glucose in NIDDM Subjects: A Criteria-Based Literature Review," *Diabetes Care* 20, no. 9: 1482–86.

15. See Goodman, *Regulation of Medical Care: Is the Price Too High?*

16. Although for the terminally ill, this is an idea worth considering.

17. Gail A. Jensen and Michael A. Morrisey, "Mandated Benefit Laws and Employer-Sponsored Health Insurance," *Health Insurance Association of America,* January 1999.

18. There is a growing literature on how to design such arrangements. See John H. Cochrane, "Time-Consistent Health Insurance," *Journal of Political Economy* 103, no. 3 (June 1995): 445–73; Mark V. Pauly, Howard Kunreuther and Richard Hirth, "Guaranteed Renewability in Insurance," *Journal of Risk and Uncertainty* 10 (March 1995): 143–56. See also Bradley Herrick and Mark Pauly, "Incentive-Compatible Guaranteed Renewable Health Insurance" NBER Working Paper 9888, National Bureau of Economic Research, July 2003; and Vip Patel and Mark V. Pauly, "Guaranteed Renewability and the Problem of Risk Variation in Individual Health Insurance Markets," *Health Affairs* (August 28, 2002) (Web exclusive).

19. What is envisioned here is a market for individual patients. For those who doubt that such a market could develop, recall that the same objection was once raised against a reinsurance market for residential housing.

20. The reason is that sellers have an incentive to charge marginal cost when no third party is involved.

21. Regina E. Herzlinger, *Market Driven Health Care: Who Wins, Who Loses in the Transformation of America's Largest Service Industry* (Reading, Mass.: Addison-Wesley, 1997), 173.

22. Harris Meyer, "Are You Ready for the Competition?" *Hospitals and Health Networks* 72, no. 7 (April 5, 1998): 25–30.

23. *New York Times Magazine,* May 3, 1998.

24. There may, however, be a legal obstacle. To our knowledge, every state government prohibits employers from buying individually owned insurance for their employees (see the discussion below) and some legal experts are convinced this practice is also outlawed under HIPAA.

25. For a fuller discussion, see John C. Goodman and Merrill Matthews, "Reforming the U.S. Health Care System," National Center for Policy Analysis," *NCPA Policy Backgrounder,* no. 149 (April 26, 1999); Pauly and Goodman, "Incremental Steps toward Health System Reform," and John C. Goodman and Gerald L. Musgrave, *Patient Power: Solving America's Health Care Crisis* (Washington, D.C.: Cato Institute, 1992), ch. 20.

Afterword

Our survey of national health insurance in countries around the world provides convincing evidence that government control of health care usually makes citizens worse off. When health care is free at the point of consumption, rationing by waiting is inevitable. Government control of the health care system makes the rationing problem worse as governments attempt to slow the use of services by limiting access to modern medical technology. Under government management, both efficiency and quality of patient care steadily deteriorate.

The lesson from other countries is that Americans would be ill-served by more government bureaucracy or more governmental control over our health care system. We need instead to limit the role of government and expand the role of the private sector and the individual in solving our health care problems.

Index

About the Authors

John C. Goodman is founder and president of the National Center for Policy Analysis, a nonprofit public policy institute with offices in Dallas, Texas, and Washington, D.C. He is the author or coauthor of more than 200 articles and seven books, including *Patient Power* (with Gerald Musgrave). He received the prestigious Duncan Black Award for the best scholarly article on public choice economics in 1988. Goodman received a Ph.D. in economics from Columbia University and has taught at a number of colleges and universities.

Gerald L. Musgrave is president of Economics America, Inc., in Ann Arbor, Michigan, and is a senior fellow with the National Center for Policy Analysis. He is the author or coauthor of more than sixty publications, including *Patient Power* (with John Goodman). He is the book review editor of *Business Economics,* and is a fellow of the National Association for Business Economics, the organization's highest honor. He also served as a presidential appointee to the National Institutes of Health Recombinant DNA Advisory Committee. Musgrave received a Ph.D. in economics from Michigan State University.

Devon M. Herrick is a senior fellow with the National Center for Policy Analysis. He has authored a number of studies on consumer-driven health care, Internet-based medicine, health insurance, and the uninsured. He also served as a research assistant at the Bruton Center for Development Studies and taught health economics at the University of Texas at Dallas. He previously worked in health care accounting and financial management for a Dallas-area health care system. Herrick received a Ph.D. in political economy from the University of Texas at Dallas.